"What every parent should know about their kids and sex. Amber's book gives moms and dads the insights we need to offer our kids advice that's relevant to their lives."

—Meredith Vieira

"A parenting book written by a twenty-six-year-old—brilliant! Comprehensive and accurate without being overwhelming, it's about the heart as well as the body."

—Katharine O'Connell White, MD, MPH, OB-GYN at Tufts University–Baystate Medical Center

"Amber is totally in touch with today's teens."

—Deborah Arrindell, Vice President, American Social Health Association

"Needed more now than ever, *Talking Sex with Your Kids* helps parents through the minefields of today's sexualized childhood. Avoiding simplistic formulae and mandates about what to do, Amber Madison uses a reader-friendly style to provide parents with the information and reassurance they need to connect meaningfully with their children, influence the lessons they learn, and promote the development of healthy, caring relationships in which sex will be a part when they grow up."

—Diane E. Levin, PhD, Professor of Education, Wheelock College; Coauthor of *So Sexy So Soon*

"Amber Madison is fast becoming the most trusted authority on modern issues of sex and sexuality and a conduit through which parents and children can talk openly about s-e-x."

—Dan Reimold, Author of *Sex and the University*

Foreword by BILL ALBERT,
Chief Program Officer, The National Campaign to Prevent Teen and Unplanned Pregnancy

TALKING SEX with your KIDS

KEEPING THEM SAFE AND YOU SANE — BY KNOWING WHAT THEY'RE REALLY THINKING

AMBER MADISON

Reviewed by Medical Advisor Katharine O'Connell White, MD, MPH

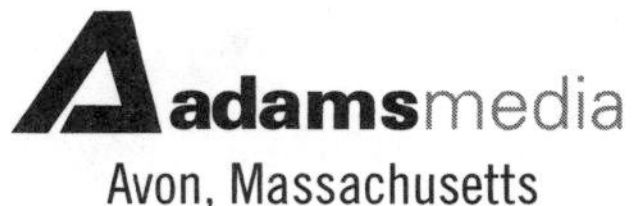

Published by
Adams Media, a division of F+W Media, Inc.
57 Littlefield Street, Avon, MA 02322. U.S.A.
www.adamsmedia.com

ISBN 10: 1-60550-662-1
ISBN 13: 978-1-60550-662-3

Printed in the United States of America.

10 9 8 7 6 5 4 3 2 1

Library of Congress Cataloging-in-Publication Data
is available from the publisher.

To Lucille S. Brown, artist, beauty,
New York Times fanatic, but most of all,
a woman with the deepest love for her family.

ACKNOWLEDGMENTS

No part of this came easy, and I'd like to thank all who helped me in the struggles along the way. To Dr. Katharine O'Connell White, who more than earned her name on the cover. To Bill Albert for his humble brilliance and enthusiastic support. And to Linda Brown for being the queen of STD knowledge.

A special thank-you to everyone I interviewed for this book: your different expertise and points of view helped me form my own: Jane Key, Dr. Robert Blum, Louise Lavin, Rabbi Charlie Buckholtz, Sarah Brown, Amy Cody, Jane Brown, Reverend David O'Leary, Dr. Gretchen Stuart, Dr. Denniz Zolnoun, and Andrew Drucker. Also to those who shared their stories with me: Steve, Laura, Ryan, and Kerry.

To everyone who physically made this book possible: Robin Straus for continuing to believe in me; my editor, Andrea Norville, for responding to any e-mail within two minutes; everyone at Adams Media for taking on this project; and to Jodi Solomon for always boosting my spirits.

Last but not least to my friends and family. To my parents, Roger Madison and Jane Leserman Madison for their constant support and encouragement. To Robert and Louisa Paushter for being my parenting role models. To my grandmothers, Lucille Brown and Grace Madison, for teaching me to be a freethinker and question authority. To Melinda Rhodebeck for teaching me tolerance and unconditional love. And to Todd Lichten, whose extraordinary work ethic has inspired me to be the same way.

CONTENTS

FOREWORD

It's an undeniable truth that as parents, we are more involved with our children than our parents were with us. From playdates to picking colleges, there are few parts of our children's lives we leave unattended and unremarked upon. As almost any teen will ruefully tell you, parents are only too willing to offer quite specific guidance and advice on any number of topics—think of the repeated admonitions we offer our children about eating right or being a careful driver.

So when it comes to important issues like sex and romantic relationships, why should we take a pass? Developing healthy relationships, understanding love and sex (and what the difference is), and avoiding unplanned pregnancy are arguably some of the most important parts of our children's lives. But when it comes to giving advice on these issues, so many of us feel dumbstruck. Meanwhile, our kids are busy learning about sex in the schoolyard, on the Internet, in the media . . . and the list goes on. The question for you is simple: Do you want to be part of that conversation or not?

Over the past decade plus, those of us who happily toil at The National Campaign to Prevent Teen and Unplanned Pregnancy have traveled coast to coast talking with countless parents, and we have noted a common lament. Most parents understand that they should be talking to their children about relationships, love, sex, and contraception, but they freely admit they don't know what to say, when to say it, or how to get the conversation started. Not to worry, Amber Madison is here to help. This book provides a playbook of practical ideas, thoughts, and scripts for you to use. Breaking down the double standard, it offers a list of topics you should talk about with your sons, as well as your daughters (telling teen girls to say "no" and teen boys to be "careful" just won't do). Amber's book offers basic information about STDs, how to address the barriers teens face when using contraception, the best way to discuss healthy relationships, and so much more. It explains that these topics are too important for a one-time talk, and should instead be thought of as an eighteen-year conversation. And at its core, this book underscores an important, powerful, and enduring truth: Parents matter. A lot.

We have not lost our kids to the influence of peers and popular culture. In fact, according to more than two decades of good social science and recent public opinion polling, just the opposite is true. Teens themselves say—are you sitting down?—parents influence their decisions about relationships and sex more than peers, partners, or the popular media culture. Who knew?

But recent data has also shown something else; that after fifteen straight years of decline, the teen birth rate is on the rise again. Now, more than ever, you have to be talking with your kids about sex, love, and relationships. As much as I wish this book was not necessary, I am delighted that one as straightforward and helpful as this one now exists. As the father of a perfect fifteen-year-old son (well, nearly perfect anyway), my only regret is that this book wasn't available for me to read and learn from four years ago. Parents, your job is clear: Start reading, then start talking. Your children are waiting.

Bill Albert
Chief Program Officer
The National Campaign to Prevent Teen
and Unplanned Pregnancy
August 2009

INTRODUCTION: YES, YOU MATTER

Parents look at teen sexuality as a blur of bare midriffs and wonder how in the world they can fit into that equation. But to the extent that we have a magic bullet, it is in parents, and strong, connected, communicative families. —**Bill Albert, Chief Program Officer, The National Campaign to Prevent Teen and Unplanned Pregnancy**

When doing research for this book I asked friends and family to share stories about their parents talking with them about sex. Over and over again I got the same answer: a story about a parent explaining what a period is. I also asked people if they got any books about sex when they were growing up. Again, they'd tell me which books they got about periods, or puberty, or how babies were made.

I didn't get it. I explicitly asked for stories about their parents talking about sex. What was the miscommunication here? Why were so many people's definition of sex a girl getting her period? The average girl gets her period when she's twelve. The average person first has sex when he or she is seventeen. Even age-wise it doesn't make sense. Then, I finally got it. Most people's parents didn't talk with them about sex—at least not beyond a woman's fertility or the fact that "the stork" doesn't deliver babies, vaginas do.

Very likely, your parents didn't talk with you much about sex either, but that doesn't mean you should make the same mistake with your own kids. Do you really want your child's sexual health information coming from the phys ed teacher with the tacky wind pants, bad attitude, and an IQ just high enough to explain the rules of dodge ball? Or would you rather have it come from their precocious friend who has a subscription to Maxim? Or perhaps, you prefer they develop attitudes about sexuality from shows like *Gossip Girl*, raunchy rap songs, and movies like *Knocked Up*. If you don't talk to your kids about sex, those may be their only options. It's up to you to educate your teens (and preteens) about sex and relationships. It's not the responsibility of their best friend, their phys ed teacher, or God forbid, MTV. As a parent, that job—tough as it may be—is yours.

But why listen to me? Perhaps you're wondering why you should take parenting advice from a twenty-five-year-old who has no kids. It's true. I don't know what it's like to talk with my teen about sex. And heck, I'm closer to being a teen than I am to having teen children. But this isn't a book about what it's like to be a parent—you know that already. This is a book about what it's like to be a teen, making decisions in today's sexual climate. And that's something I do know about.

To me, the most frustrating thing about being a teen was feeling like no one listened, or took you seriously. I constantly felt brushed off as an impulsive, incompetent ball of hormones, when in reality, I really did care about making good choices. In order for you and your kids to have productive conversations about sex, first you have to understand what's really going on: what they're thinking, how they feeling, and their attitudes about sex and relationships. And for your comfort and theirs, it's important for you to communicate with them about these issues in a non-psychobabble, realistic way. I've written this book to make sure that teens' voices are accounted for, as opposed to an all-adult conversation about "the teen sex crisis." It's about why teens don't always make the best decisions, what they *really* think about sex, and the kind of advice that will actually help them make better choices. Think of me not as a fellow parent, or as a peer of your teen, but as someone in the middle. I'm old enough to sit at the adult table and empathize, but still young enough to sit at the kids table and "get it."

No Really, You Matter

In the past four years while touring college campuses speaking with teens about sexuality and relationships, I've heard the same thing time and again: "Nobody has ever talked to me about this before." And that isn't something students report happily. Teens want to know more about sex, and they want to be able to go to their parents with questions and for guidance. Eighty-seven percent of teens say that it would be easier for them to postpone sexual activity and avoid pregnancy if they were able to have more open and honest conversations with their parents (The National Campaign to Prevent Teen and Unplanned Pregnancy 2007).

Many parents think that teens' friends most influence their decision to have sex. But that's not the case. It's not their friends, the media, or even their partner that plays the biggest role in teens' sexual decision making. It's you, their parents. Almost half of teens say their parents *most* influence their decision to have sex. The younger a teen is, the more influential parents are—59 percent of teens age twelve to fourteen say their parents have the most influence over their sexual decisions (The National Campaign to Prevent Teen and Unplanned Pregnancy 2007). So yes, you do make a difference.

But talking to your kids is the only way to make that difference. We've all seen the parents who try to avoid conversations about sex by setting early curfews, draconian dating rules, or threatening to fit their daughters for chastity belts. And none of those approaches work. If teens are dead set on having sex, they'll find a way to make it happen, with or without your consent. You can't always control what your kids do, but you can greatly influence how they think.

Will talking about sex be uncomfortable? At times. Intimidating? Probably. "Totally gross" to your teen? It's a possibility. Maybe you worry about feeling embarrassed, or that saying anything at all will encourage sexual activity (though, rest assured, decades of research supports the fact that it won't). Most likely, you have no idea what to say or how to say it, or you don't feel like you know enough about sex yourself. But the reality is, you're already equipped with everything you need to talk with your kids about sex; it's just a matter of jumping over your own mental hurdles.

Take comfort in the fact that even with as little as you may know now, you can still be a tremendous resource for your kids. The most important thing you can do for your children's sexual health is to make them feel good about themselves, let them know you care about them and that you want to be there to help. And that's not something you have to learn from a book.

What you will learn from this book is what teens are really thinking about sex, sexuality, and relationships, and how to help them make the healthiest choices. You'll get a basic understanding of sexual health topics ranging from which STDs one can contract from which sexual activities to how emergency contraception works and when a girl should use it. You'll learn how to talk with your kids about sex, when to bring it up, and what to say. You'll also learn to find the line between being an open parent and being unnecessarily graphic and giving *too much* information. This book will help you get out of your own way—get over your embarrassment, challenge your misconceptions, and arm you with all the information you need to help your children make informed choices about birth control and STD prevention and think critically about their sexual decisions.

Teens aren't the inherently irresponsible beings they're so often made out to be. They want to make informed choices about sex—but if they aren't given information or guidance, the reality is they'll make choices anyway. As parents, you too have a choice. You can let your teens venture into the sexual world unguided. Or you can start an open, honest, and realistic dialogue about sex and relationships.

Talking Tips Throughout This Book

As you read through the rest of this book you'll notice many sections entitled, "Real Life Advice." These quotes are suggestions for how you may want to phrase a certain topic using words that will feel natural and arguments that will seem relevant to your teen.

You'll also notice other sections: the "TMI Warning" boxes. These "Too Much Information Warnings" are to help you understand what is best left out of a parent-child sex talk. It's possible to be *too* open with your kids, and these will alert you to when you're crossing that line.

POP QUIZ: ARE YOU AN ASKABLE PARENT?

1. **Your teen asks you if you can get STDs from having oral sex. You say:**
   A. "Why? Are you having oral sex?"
   B. "I think so. But I'm not sure which ones. Let me look into it and get back to you."
   C. "I'm not a doctor, how should I know?"

2. **You find out that a few freshmen at your teen's high school have been caught having sex in the bathroom. You:**
   A. Tell your kids, "Good thing that wasn't you or you'd be grounded for life."
   B. Talk with your teen about the right reasons to have sex and the type of relationships where sex is appropriate.
   C. Hope your child isn't having sex.

3. **You're eating dinner one night when your fifteen-year-old daughter says, "I'm done with boys; they're such jerks! From now on, Sarah's my lesbian lover." You say:**
   A. "That's not dinner-table conversation!"
   B. "Honey, figuring out your sexuality is a little more complicated than being upset with a guy."
   C. Kids say the darnedest things, you ignore her outburst. "Honey, can you hand me a napkin."

4. **Labia. Your first thought is:**
   A. I can't believe I'm reading a book with the word "labia" in it.
   B. My child's second word.
   C. Did I plant those in my garden?

5. **Your teenage son asks you if a girl can get pregnant on her period. You:**
   - **A.** Freak out. Not only is he having sex, he's gotten a girl pregnant!
   - **B.** Are happy he's asking questions about sex and pregnancy.
   - **C.** Are surprised he knows what a period is.

6. **You go out to a family movie and there's an unexpected lengthy sex scene. You:**
   - **A.** Grab your teens firmly by the hand, and walk them out of the theater.
   - **B.** Later that night talk with your kids about how unrealistic it is that characters rarely talk about condom use when sex is portrayed in movies.
   - **C.** Later that night yell at your spouse for picking out a PG-13 family movie.

Mostly A's:

Go to a quiet place with this book and start reading. Go directly to this place. Do not pass go; do not collect $200. When you're done reading, start trying to create a more open and judgment-free atmosphere in your house. Talking with your kids about sexual health issues, relationships, and sexual decision-making is different than telling them to go off and have sex. STDs are everywhere, unplanned pregnancies happen every day, and teens make sexual choices they regret. If you want to help your teens avoid the negative consequences that can come as a result of having sex, you have to talk with them about sexual issues—and telling them to "just say no" doesn't count as talking.

Mostly B's:

It's great that you are so open with your kids about sex. Difficult sexual issues are going to be much easier for you and your kids to talk about because sex isn't a taboo topic in your house. Do remember, however, that sex is an embarrassing issue for many teens, and it's important to be sensitive to that. Even though you may think talking about sex is no big deal, bringing up sexual issues in the middle of a family get-together or around a group of your teen's friends could be humiliating for your child. As great as it is that you're comfortable with sexual topics, always keep in mind that your child probably isn't at that comfort level yet. Now all you need is to know what to say.

Mostly C's:

Hey you! Yes, you! Get your head out of the clouds. Your teen is thinking about sex, even if he or she isn't doing it. Choosing to stay out of your kids' private lives isn't helping them at all. I'm not saying you have to get all up in their business, but you should have a general idea of what's going on. Start talking to your kids. Talk to them about all sorts of issues, and eventually start broaching topics that have to do with sex and relationships. It may be a little uncomfortable for you to talk about those issues, but it's part of your parental duty. And what's a little embarrassment when your child's physical and emotional health is at stake?

Chapter One
THE WAY THINGS STAND

I'm a believer in prevention. Your chances are always better when you work on problems on the front end. Anticipate future issues and work to prevent them from happening.

—Jane Key, sexual violence services coordinator, South Carolina Department of Health

Like staring at a giant mess, you're probably a little overwhelmed about where to start with the whole sex talk thing. Also like a giant mess, it's best to know exactly what you're dealing with before you dive in. Think of this chapter as the before picture: how teens are acting, what they're doing, what they're being taught in school, and the values you've already instilled in them that will make sex talks easier. As you'll see, there is a bit of a disaster zone as far as teens and sex are concerned. But just like the party they'll throw when you go out of town—with enough effort, it can be cleaned up.

Twelve Going on Twenty

As I've witnessed on the faces of many shocked parents, there are few things more frightening than your kids starting to act overtly sexual. Maybe they dress provocatively, are constantly talking about the opposite sex, seem obsessed with racy jokes, or talk like they're experienced. I cannot tell you how many parents come to me concerned about the dirty dancing at bar mitzvah parties, the lacy thongs their daughter got as a birthday present, or their son making constant references to oral sex. Parents worry that the way their kids are acting is an indication that they're looking for sex, are about to have sex, or think sex isn't a big deal. But much of the time there is a disconnect between the sexual image adolescents might project and how they actually feel about sex. Culturally, sex jokes are everywhere, and teens know they're taboo. They also know how people act on TV and in movies and that sex sells (or at least gets people to pay attention). When teens start acting and dressing sexually, they're often just imitating their friends, pushing the envelope, or trying to show off.

One summer, my friend's twelve-year-old brother called her from camp and said, "Hold on, I gotta go; I'm about to get laid." After freaking out, and calling him back to ask what he meant by "get laid," he clarified, "there's a girl here I like and I was going over to talk to her." Apparently, either he was misinformed about what "get laid" meant, or he just thought "get laid" had a cooler ring to it than "eating lunch with." Either way, what he was saying didn't match up at all with what he was doing.

Sometimes teens just don't get it. They may look like adults, but their minds are a bit more innocent. When thirteen-year-old girls walk around in tight shirts with half their breasts exposed, they're probably thinking something along the lines of: "Sweet, look what just grew on my chest." Or they're proud to look like Megan Fox, Blake Lively, or some other hot celeb on the cover of *Seventeen*. What they probably aren't thinking is, "I need to get laid, maybe this shirt will do the trick."

I'm not trying to convince you that your young teens won't actually have sex; some will, way too soon. What I want to do is encourage you to look past the yoga pants, pelvic thrusting, and sexual dialogue, and remember that beneath all that crap is a confused, vulnerable kid. A kid who still thinks sex is a big deal. One who may act like he or she knows everything, but still has questions, needs your guidance, and will be influenced by what you say. So take a deep breath. Don't freak out thinking that your young kids are having sex just because they may be acting a bit sexual, but do take it as a sign that at the very least sex is on their minds. Perhaps, the way your kids are acting is their subconscious way of encouraging you to initiate the conversation.

How Many Are Actually Doing It, and Does It Really Matter?

While many kids are just talking about sex, or acting sexually, some *are* actually doing it. According to the 2007 Youth Risk Behavior Survey, by freshman year of high school, one out of every three students has had sex. And by senior year of high school, that proportion rises to nearly two out of three. Some sexually active teens have only had sex with a long-term girlfriend or boyfriend, but others are being less selective about their choices—roughly one-fifth of high school seniors have had sex with four or more partners. What's most concerning, though, is the fact that many teens who are having sex are doing it without protection. Less than two-thirds of sexually active high school students used a condom the last time they had sex, and less than one-sixth used birth control pills. In nonnumeric terms, many high school students are having sex, and many of them are having sex without protection. And these are not inflated statistics from inner-city populations. This is happening everywhere, in middle-class and upscale neighborhoods too.

HOW DOES THE UNITED STATES MEASURE UP?
We have the highest teen pregnancy and STD rate of any country in the industrialized world. Source: United Nations Statistics Division 2006 and American Social Health Association 2006.

Unprotected teen sex is a huge problem. It's a problem because nearly one-third of American women get pregnant before they turn twenty (The National Campaign to Prevent Teen and Unplanned Pregnancy). Those girls then have to make the difficult decision of becoming teen mothers (and likely dropping out of high school or college), having an abortion, or choosing adoption. Unprotected sex also means STDs. And as most recently measured by the American Social Health Association, by age twenty-five, half of all young people in this country will have contracted some sort of STD. Some of those people will get lucky and get a curable STD that they detect right away. Some will contract a curable STD but not discover they have it until after it has caused irreversible damage to their reproductive system. Others will contract viruses that will stay in their bodies for the rest of their lives. And all these physical repercussions speak nothing of the emotional turmoil caused by having sex in the wrong situations.

I'm not bringing this up to scare you, but to point out that ultimately your concern for your children's emotional and physical health may be the key to trumping any unease you have about talking to them about sex. Discovering one's sexuality has the potential to be a positive and healthy part of becoming an adult, and you can help ensure that for your child it is. With the right guidance, teens are much more likely to make sexual decisions that will not result in an STD, an unwanted pregnancy, or emotional distress.

Where Are the Schools in All This?

You would hope that with stats like the ones just mentioned, public schools would be stepping up to the plate to help. And many do step up. They just don't all help.

The majority of school districts have a policy to teach sex education. But over a third of public school districts nationwide—and half of public school districts in the South—have a policy to teach *abstinence-only* sex education (Guttmacher Institute 2006). For those of you who aren't already aware of this approach, abstinence-only programs teach that the *only* way to avoid getting pregnant or getting an STD is to avoid having sex. Although these programs include discussions of healthy relationships and setting limits, they don't discuss condoms or other birth control choices other than to emphasize their failure rates. The shared goal of most abstinence-only programs is to convince teens to remain virgins. (Of course, one of the inherent problems with this idea is that teens can still get STDs from sexual activities they don't consider to affect their status as a virgin.)

As you may have guessed, the message of "no sex before marriage" often doesn't stick. As research has consistently found, teens in abstinence-only programs aren't any less likely to have sex (Kirby 2007). Then, when those teens do have sex, they do so without ever being formally educated about condoms, birth control, or sexual decision-making.

Many schools reject abstinence-only programs and take a more realistic approach. They follow the recommendations of the American Academy of Pediatrics, American College of Obstetricians and Gynecologists, American Medical Association, American Public Health Association, and many others, and teach students about contraception as well as abstinence. And it's these types of comprehensive sex education programs that have actually been shown to delay sexual activity. But most important, when teens who have gone through these programs do have sex, they are more likely to use condoms and less likely to sleep with many different partners (Alford 2008). If your child's school doesn't offer a comprehensive sex education program, you may want to look into other groups in your community that do.

Best-case scenario, your children have been lucky enough to get some type of worthwhile sex education. But that doesn't mean you're off the hook. Even teens who are taught about the nuts and bolts of safer sex probably don't get all of their questions answered by their school sex ed class. When I talk to young adults, I often get asked questions that have more to do with emotional concerns than physical acts. Teens wonder: "How can I feel less awkward about using a condom?" "What do I say if my partner doesn't like them?" and "Will taking birth control pills make me fat?" More generally, many simply want to know: "When is it a good idea to have sex?" or "How do I know I'm in a good relationship?" Both the young men and young women I talk with tell me they've had sexual experiences they feel good about, and sexual experiences they wish they could take back. But even after reflecting on their encounters, many need guidance to understand which situations lead to positive experiences and which situations lead to negative ones.

One-size-fits-all sex ed classes will never be able to replace the advice and guidance that a parent can give. Classes don't give feedback when it looks like a teen might be in an unhealthy relationship, or provide someone a teen can go to whenever a question or concern might arise. They don't convince teens that they're worthy of respect or to never settle for a relationship in which they're being treated unfairly. Regardless of who else is talking to your kids about sex, there is always some kind of support that only you will be able to offer.

Why Teens Don't Just Come to You

In an ideal world, if your teens had questions about sex, they'd just walk right up to you and ask. Unfortunately, many teens feel like they can't go to their parents for sexual guidance. Eighty-three percent of teens won't initiate conversations about sex because they worry about their parents' reaction (Kaiser Family Foundation 2002). Most worry that if they ask their parents about sex, their parents will automatically assume they're sexually active and get mad. And honestly, I don't think that's an illegitimate fear.

I had a friend in high school who was grounded for months because her parents found the birth control pills she hid under her bed. And just recently a father said to me, "I've got one answer to my kid's questions about sex: 'Don't do it.'" Out of fear and discomfort over the idea of their children becoming sexually active, many parents' unchecked emotional reaction is simply anger. But getting angry at the thought of your teens having sex isn't going to help them make responsible sexual choices—it will just confirm their suspicions that they can't come to you for guidance.

Even if teens aren't worried about their parents' reaction, many don't initiate sex talks because they're embarrassed or they don't know how to bring it up. Ironically, two of the same reasons you may not be talking to your teen. But at the end of the day, one of you is going to have to get over it—and as the parent, that burden falls on you. But don't worry; as intimidated as you may be to approach your children about sex, the truth is, you've already laid the groundwork for the values that will see them through even their toughest sexual decisions.

The Values Your Kids (Hopefully) Have Already

Many of the skills teens need to be able to make good sexual choices don't have to do with sex at all. And in fact, they're the same general skills that should keep your kids away from drugs, academic ambivalence, and other destructive behaviors. The following are the good values you have already started cultivating in your teen and should continue to help develop. If these aren't values you've already instilled, it's never too late to start.

Good Self-Esteem

In order to make wise sexual choices, your children need to feel good about themselves. Having confidence and a strong sense of self-worth can be a difficult thing to build, especially for young adults. Many people I know look back on high school as the most insecure period of their lives. But as a parent, there is a lot you can do to help. Here are the things that you can do to help your children feel good about themselves their whole lives:

- **Encourage their interest in hobbies and extracurricular activities.** Jane Key, the sexual violence service coordinator for the South Carolina Department of Health, suggests that parents can help build their children's self-esteem by "looking at what they are interested in and what they do well, and encouraging them to nurture that." Not every child is going to be a star athlete, a straight-A student, or the prom queen. But everyone is good at something, or interested enough in something to want to become decent at it. It is possible that that talent or interest will take some trial and error to find. This is not to say you should be that type of obnoxious parent that makes a kid go to soccer, karate, piano, Spanish lessons, and ballroom dancing all at once—but encourage your kids to try different things until they find one that sticks. No matter what kids' school life is like, having a few hours a week where they are truly in their element will help them feel good about themselves in their day-to-day life.

- **Help them see the positive.** Kids are going to mess up, and they're going to discover their flaws. That is inevitable. But you can help soften the blow of their faults by giving them positive feedback and helping them see the silver lining of the negative things that happen to them. Take your kids' focus away from what they don't like: "That bully only makes fun of you because you're so much smarter than he is. Your smarts will get you ahead, and his attitude is just going to hold him back." Or, "It's not the end of the world you bombed that geometry test. All in all you're a great student. This bad score is just a sign that maybe you should get some extra help from your teacher."
- **Show them—and tell them—they are loved.** After my dad would tuck me in at night, he'd always make me repeat "the two most important things." Now, as an adult, he writes them in any cards or e-mails he sends me. The two things he tells me constantly are: "I've always enjoyed every age I've ever been," and "You know we love you very much." Sex educators, doctors, therapists, and researchers can all agree on this: your children need to be constantly reminded that you love them unconditionally. Even when you're upset with them, even when you're having a bad

day, and even when they act like they hate you. How you remind them is up to you, but letting them know they are loveable will be central to their feelings of self-worth.

If you haven't always made a constant effort to raise your children's self-esteem you can always start now. Self-confidence is a constant struggle, and likely something your kids will need help with throughout the course of their life.

Respect for Their Bodies and Other People's Bodies

Kids need to feel good about their bodies before you can expect them to have healthy sexual relationships. And by bodies, I don't just mean their figures, I mean their genitals—penises and vaginas, folks. If you send messages to your kids that imply their bodies are shameful, gross, dirty, and embarrassing, and that it's abnormal for them to touch or look at themselves, you're undermining messages you're going to want to send them later. A basic building block of good sexual health is encouraging your kids to take care of their bodies and be conscious of what they do with them. Because of that, you have to teach your kids their bodies are something that's worthy of respect. If their genitals are filthy, shameful places anyway, what's the point of taking care of them?

Part of teaching children to feel good about and respect their bodies is teaching them boundaries. The first time I worked as a mother's helper, the woman I was working for had to remind her son, "It's not appropriate to play with your penis at the dinner table." Although now your kids may be old enough to realize touching themselves is a private activity, you may still have to do some regulating on your son's new favorite comeback, "suck it" ("That's not an okay thing for you to be saying, and it probably makes people uncomfortable"), or your daughter trying to leave the house wearing little more than a bikini ("Honey, what type of message do you think that's sending?").

You should also make sure your kids understand they have to respect other people's bodies too. It's not okay to touch people without their permission, and likewise it's not okay for other people to touch them without permission. (Obviously, you're going to have to differentiate between a friendly hug and more sexual touching.) If your kids have learned to value other people's bodies as well as their own, you have set them up to make considerate and responsible sexual choices when they are older.

The Confidence to Question Authority

This advice may seem a bit counterintuitive, as you probably don't want little revolutionaries running around challenging everything you say. But in the interest of your children's sexual health, you don't want them to be completely obedient and submissive either. "Respecting authority is not always the best idea in all situations," says Robert Blum, MD, MPH, PhD, director of Johns Hopkins Urban Health Institute. "Parents need to give their children the clear message: I matter, I'm important, and just because you say it's so doesn't mean it's so." One day, your children probably will be in situations (sexual or otherwise) where they are going to have to assert themselves and stand up to a teacher, a boss, an older relative, an older sex partner, or a popular friend. In those situations, kids need to know the people in control aren't always right, and that they shouldn't *always* do what they're told.

When your kids start engaging in sexual activities, they're probably going to be engaging in those activities with people they respect, have crushes on, are popular, good looking, or for whatever other reason seem like they are in a position of authority. In order for your teens to be able to respect their own boundaries, they have to know that just because someone with power wants them to do something, it doesn't mean they are obligated to do it; their own feelings matter just as much. Clearly, you don't want to teach your kids to be arrogant, but encouraging a manageable attitude of "no one pushes me around," will serve your kids well as they start to enter sexual relationships (especially your daughters).

What You Should Work On as a Parent

Just as the values you've instilled in your children play a role in their sexual health, the type of parent you've been will play a role in how your sex talks are received. The following sections are about behaviors *you* should change in order to have the most productive conversations with your children.

Be a Role Model

Before kids know any better, they just assume everyone's family life is like their own. They look at their mom and form opinions about women, look at their dad and form opinions about men, and look at the way their parents interact and form opinions about love. Kids' parents' relationships serve as their most intimate example of what a romantic relationship is supposed to look like. If you and your spouse are kind and loving toward each other (at least in front of your kids), that's the behavior they're going to learn. If you're always yelling at each other or putting one another down, that's what they'll learn. It's no secret that kids who grow up in a family where there is physical or emotional abuse are likely to repeat that pattern within their own relationships. As a parent, you should be mirroring the type of relationship you would want for your children.

Kids also look to their parents for examples of sex roles within a relationship. If mom is always allowing dad to boss her around, her daughter is going to learn to be passive, and her son is going to think he should be the one who calls all the shots. If dad is emotionally withdrawn and unavailable, his son is going to learn to be the same way, and his daughter will be less likely to seek out emotionally supportive partners. When I asked Robert Blum about concerns of gender stereotypes in the media, he told me, "More than anything, kids learn stereotypes from how their parents interact." With the limited experience I've had around younger kids, this didn't surprise me. If there's one thing I know about children, it's that they really do pick up on *everything*. They're always listening—even when you're not talking to them.

This is not to say that your children are doomed if your relationship with your spouse isn't perfect; no one's relationship is. But you can make an effort to always act respectfully toward each other whenever your kids are in earshot (even if you are divorced). And although you may not be able to show your kids what a healthy relationship looks like, you can certainly speak with them about it. Don't be afraid to admit the faults in your relationship, and teach your children to avoid those faults in their own.

Be an Available Parent

If you haven't always made time for your kids, you can't waltz in to talk with them about sex and expect that they'll listen. They'll think: "Oh, so now you want to talk? Screw off." If you've been an absent parent, before you try to dish out advice or influence their decisions, you need to form a real relationship with your kids. Otherwise, your words carry no weight. Spend time with them during the week or on the weekends doing an activity they enjoy. Make an effort to share meals with them, ask them about their day, and go to their sporting events or after-school activities.

If you are involved in your children's lives, congratulations, that's 90 percent of the battle right there. What you need to do now is give your relationship some credit. Your kids love you, they respect you, they value your opinion, and they want to make you proud. So the things you tell them matter.

Talking with your kids about sex may not be easy. But where there's a will there's a way. Knowing that you can greatly influence your children's emotional and physical health—that's your will. Your way—that's Chapter 2.

Chapter Two
HOW TO TALK TO YOUR TEEN ABOUT SEX

I was thirteen and my father was driving my brother and me to a Smashing Pumpkins concert when mid-trip he turned off the stereo. "My father never gave me this talk, and I promised not to make the same mistake with my sons." He told us about his own misguided puberty. Many unnecessary anecdotes led into his main point: it was "only natural" and that we should feel free to ask him if we were unsure of anything.

—Ryan, age twenty-six

Getting a colonoscopy, swimming laps in a freezing lake, and having a group dinner with everyone you've ever dated are probably all options that seem more comfortable than talking with your kids about sex. I get it, talking to your kids about sex feels awkward. You may worry about embarrassing yourself, embarrassing them, and sitting down for twenty minutes of general misery. And it's okay if you feel this way—many parents do.

Even if you've been able to be open with your kids about their body parts, and answer their general questions about "where babies come from," it's a different ball game when you're talking to your kids about sex in the context of, "you may be doing this soon." But just like most people don't have their first kiss, first relationship, and lose their virginity all at once, you don't have to jump right in with conversations about sexual intercourse. You can take a gradual approach and lead up to it by talking about other sexual issues first.

The good news is: you shouldn't have one huge conversation about anything and everything sexual that's your only shot at imparting sexual values to your teen. You should have dozens of conversations, hundreds of them, as many as you need. So if your first few runs don't go that well, it's not a big deal—you have plenty of time to make up for them. Your sex talks don't have to be drawn-out sessions either; they can be short pearls of wisdom, or brief conversations. And they don't even have to be premeditated or planned out. You can say something when the mood hits, when it comes up naturally, or at a time you and your teen are really getting along.

There are many tricks for making your sex talks less nerve-racking. This chapter is about learning those tricks, getting out of your own way, and understanding how to talk with your kids about sex in a productive way.

Getting Over Your Own Embarrassment

Penis. Say it out loud. Vagina. Say that too. Sex. Say it. If you're blushing, sweating, or just said the words in your head, say them again, louder. And again, and again, until you've said them so many times that the words no longer have meaning. When those get easy, try "oral sex," "anal sex," and "vaginal lubrication."

I'm sure this exercise seems ridiculous to some of you, and maybe even raunchy to others, but I promise, it will help. The more you say sexual words, the more immune to them you get. You start to see through the hype, shock, and horror, and realize that saying them isn't going to set off any type of earth-shattering reaction. They are just words, describing body parts, bodily functions, and humans' natural inclination to reproduce. They are just words, that yes, you can even say in front of your children. And the more comfortable you become with these words, the easier it will be to speak with your children about sex.

Sex is hard to talk about only because we've learned it should be. But it's completely possible to unlearn the discomfort our society has associated with sexuality. Before your kids were born, the idea of changing diapers was probably somewhat horrifying as well. But after changing your fiftieth diaper, you were likely pretty numb to it. You *can* get over your embarrassment about sex; it's just going to mean taking the time to think about it, talk about it, and realize it's not a topic that's inherently humiliating.

Worst-case scenario, no matter what you do, you still feel completely embarrassed about talking to your kids about sex. And in that case, tough shit. As Jerusalem-based rabbi Charlie Buckholtz explains, "Certain things where the stakes are so high, embarrassment is a nonissue. You're not children; you're parents. Grow up! Not talking to your kids about sex is real negligence that leads to real consequences." With time, talking about sex should get much easier. But even if it doesn't, that's okay too. A little awkwardness has never killed anyone; bad sexual choices, on the other hand, might.

Setting the Tone

When you talk to your children about sex, you set the tone. If you can walk into a sex talk calm and collected and talk about the issues seemingly unfazed, then it's going to be a much more comfortable experience for both you and your child. The more relaxed your conversations are, the more often they will happen, because it won't be something the two of you dread.

Calm and Collected

There are two approaches you can take to make your conversations more comfortable. The first approach is to play it cool and remain calm even if on the inside you're on the verge of a panic attack. As a Latin teacher of mine used to say, "Fake it till you make it." Isn't that what parenting is about anyway, pretending you know what you're doing?

If you're planning to bring up a conversation later that day, go over your thoughts in your head, and plan out what you're going to say. Think about how you would discuss the importance of hand washing, why it's wrong to steal, or any other nonsexual topic, and try to mirror that tone. Then, when you're actually talking to your teen, relax your shoulders, keep your hands in one place, and if your child is right in front of you, look him or her in the eye. Try not to talk too quickly, repeatedly clear your throat, or say lots of "ums." As the talk goes on, you'll become more comfortable anyway, and by the end, you probably won't even be faking it.

As a kid, it's hard to understand that your parents are people too. This means your child may not instinctively think you would feel embarrassed talking about sex. The majority of kids assume their parents know what they're doing and have everything under control (it's not until much later we realize you learned as you went). Use your child's naïveté to your advantage—if you don't give your teens a reason to think you're uncomfortable, they probably won't.

Acknowledge the Awkwardness

If you know you're extremely uncomfortable, or just aren't a good actor, playing it cool probably won't work. Your second option is to acknowledge the awkwardness of the situation at the beginning. To do that, start the conversation with something like, "This is embarrassing for me to talk about, and it might be embarrassing for you too. But these are such important issues we need to talk about them anyway." Recognizing the discomfort that can result from talking about sex gives your teens (and you) license to feel nervous, and reassurance that it's okay if they do. It also, in a sense, takes the elephant out of the room. Once you acknowledge the awkwardness, you can move on—as opposed to it overshadowing the entire conversation.

If you do take this approach, the only caution I would give is to make clear that you're completely okay talking about uncomfortable issues. You don't want to give off the impression that you don't really want to be having this talk but are doing it out of parental obligation. Your goal should be to get across that you're always happy to talk about difficult issues, even if it is embarrassing.

When to Bring It Up

First of all, scratch the idea of one big sex talk you have when your child gets his or her first real girlfriend or boyfriend. No one wants that. Not you, not your child, and not sex education experts. There's no way you can cover everything in one sit down conversation, and as your child gets older and moves through different relationships, the questions and concerns will change anyway.

Instead of waiting for your teens to ask you questions, or looking for signs they may soon become sexually active, just assume that sex is something they have on their minds. Bill Albert, the chief program officer of The National Campaign to Prevent Teen and Unplanned Pregnancy tells parents this, "The median age at which kids first have sex is seventeen, and that has remained pretty stable over the years. But there are precious few fourteen-year-olds who aren't thinking about it. Assume it's a natural part of growing up." If you are the parent of an adolescent, he or she is thinking about sex—whether or not they are planning on doing it in the near future. So instead of waiting until the last second and throwing condoms at them as they walk out the door to their senior prom, start talking to them now.

Remember, sex isn't just intercourse. Many of the negative consequences (both physical and emotional) that can come from careless decisions about intercourse can come from careless decisions about other sex acts as well. Certainly by high school I would guess that a good number of kids have had a crush, maybe gone on a pseudo-date, French kissed someone, or even gone further. Something as seemingly innocent as an eighth-grade crush could be an opportunity for you to start talking with your child about unrequited love and start building trust around issues of romantic relationships and sexual activity. Every kid is different, but if I had to pin down an age, I'd say toward the end of middle school and the beginning of high school is the time to start talking to your kids about more tangible sexual issues (condom use, contraception, STDs, and sexual decision making).

If you're going to overshoot it one way or the other, it's better to talk with your kids a little too early than it is to talk with them a little too late. You don't want to start having conversations about sex when you think they're having sex, you want to start having those conversations *before* they do it. Many topics will be easier to talk about when they're a little younger anyway. They may not have thought about sex in much detail yet, and you can catch them before they've started to form definite opinions. It will always be easier to shape their opinion on something than it will be to change it once it's solidified.

How to Bring It Up

Sitting down, face to face, with the intention of having a talk—regardless of what the talk is about—is an intimidating situation. There is no reason why you need to be talking to your teen about sex in that sort of a setting. Talking to your teen in a more natural environment will likely be much easier for both of you. The following are some times you might consider talking about sex:

- **While in the car** (when you expect that you will be there for a while). One of the best times to bring up a sex talk is the car. Not only can your teen not get up and run away, but neither can you. You don't have to worry about any interruptions, and for better or worse, the two of you are stuck.

An added bonus of talking to your teen while in the car is that you have the perfect excuse to avoid eye contact. If you were talking to your teen in another setting, and avoided eye contact all together it would seem odd. In the car, you need to be watching the road, and not making eye contact is completely normal. If you're feeling really squeamish about bringing up sexual issues, talking about it while driving may be a good option. Just make sure you're still paying at least *some* attention to the road.

- **While on a walk.** If you start talking to your teen about sex while you're on a walk, the perspiration on your forehead has a chance of passing as normal. Talking while walking can create a nice leisurely pace for the conversation. There's not as much of a rush to fill pauses because you're not just sitting there in an awkward silence, you're still walking. This allows both you and your teen to take time to think carefully about what to say.

Talking while walking also allows you to make eye contact when you want to, and look away at times you don't. Using the "let's take a walk" approach is good for active people who enjoy being outdoors (not the best option if your teen is a mall rat and hates being outside). It may also be a good idea if you expect the talk to be particularly tense or suspect strong emotional reactions, since being out in nature may have a calming effect on both of you.

- **While cooking, cleaning, fishing, bowling, shooting hoops, at the zoo, etc.** Bringing up the issue of sex while you're in the middle of an activity will take pressure off of the conversation because you'll be doing two things at once. "Do you worry about being able to use a condom? Oh wow, look at that chimp." "You know that you can get STDs from oral sex, right? Damn, nice shot!" Because your talk will be interspersed with conversations about the activity you are doing, it will feel less intense.

Some words of caution, however: If you are going to bring up the issue of sex in a public place, make sure that you do have some degree of privacy. One thing that that your teen really doesn't want is to have to listen to you talk about sex while others are in earshot. So while an activity may be a good distraction, make sure you are far enough away from other people that it remains an A-B conversation. (To ensure greater privacy, you may want to visit an attraction on an off day, like a weekday morning.)

- **When you can't see each other.** If you aren't naturally good at confrontation, or your teen is very shy, it might be to your advantage to talk about sex at times when the two of you can't see each other. I spoke with one parent recently who told me she used to read a puberty book to her daughter while her daughter was in the shower. Even though they were in the same room and could easily talk, they were divided by the shower curtain and didn't have to look at each other.

Wherever you bring up the topic of sex, make sure that you leave adequate time for the conversation, that it's unlikely you'll be interrupted by anyone, and that you're somewhere both you and your teen feel comfortable. Also be sure that it's not just a one-way street—ask your child if he or she has any thoughts or questions when you're done. Even if there is no response right away, let your request hang for a bit before leaving the room or changing the subject. Always end any talk you have by reiterating that you're happy to answer any questions your teen has, or to talk about any sex or relationship issues that might be on his or her mind.

Ways of Starting the Conversation

Getting yourself to utter the words "I want to talk to you about sex" will probably be more difficult than the actual conversation that follows. Saying that first line is half the battle. So what is a good opening line?

As an overarching rule, I'd say keep the psychobabble on the bookshelf. Unless you work in the health care field and it is your natural way of talking, scratch the idea of using phrases like, "I've noticed you're developing and I think it's time we initiate a dialogue about sexual intercourse." "Noticed you're developing," what does that even mean? Developing what exactly? Why dance around the issue with big words? If what you are saying to your teen isn't something that would naturally come out of your mouth, it's going to make the situation even more uncomfortable because you won't be acting like yourself.

When choosing how to start a conversation about sex, say something direct, and something that sounds like you. From there, you can segue into whatever topic you want to talk about. Following are some suggestions of lines you might want to use to initiate a conversation about sex:

> "'Lick you like a lollipop,' that's kind of sexual to be on the radio, don't you think? Do people your age consider oral sex to be a big deal?"

> "I hope you're not too uncomfortable talking with me about this, but I'd like to talk with you about when sex is a good idea."

> "I want you to know that if you ever have any questions about sex, I'm here to answer them for you. You might be wondering . . . ."

> "I was thinking the other day, has anyone ever showed you how to use a condom?"

> "I don't know if you or any of your friends are considering having sex, but there are so many things to think about before becoming sexually active."

"So yesterday I started thinking about how little I was told about dating and relationships as a kid, and I want you to be better prepared than I was."

"You know I love you and never want to see you hurt. So even though it might be uncomfortable, I really want us to start talking about sex."

"It's funny how when they show sex scenes in movies, they hardly ever talk about or show any kind of condom use. That's so unrealistic. With all of the STDs out there!"

"Did your health class talk about STDs at all?"

"Obviously this would have killed the plot of the movie, but Juno seemed like a smart girl, don't you think she would have gotten on birth control pills before having sex?"

General Talking Tips

Although bringing up the issue of sex may be half the battle, the other half is actually having the conversation. The following are some general tips to follow when talking with your kids about any sexual issue.

Talk Your Age

When talking to your kids about sex, use terms like "penis" and "vagina." They're medically accurate, matter-of-fact words that you should get used to saying in front of your kids. If your kids are old enough to be thinking about sex, they're old enough to be talked to like adults. Don't patronize them by talking to them about their "privates," their "thingies," or their "special places." On the other hand, don't overdo it by using their lingo.

Your job is to be a parent, not a friend. No one wants to hear their parents talk about cocks, pussies, or dicks.

It also doesn't work to try to avoid referring to genitalia or sex acts all together. Trying to avoid using explicit terms will make you look uncomfortable, and make the conversation more painful. You shouldn't be explaining condom use by saying, "It's important that you roll the condom down your . . . you know . . . before you start to . . . ahemmmm." Show your kids that talking about sex acts and body parts is a natural and necessary conversation by being straightforward and scientific.

Use the Media

Sex is in the media all the time—be it in a song, a movie, a TV show, a commercial, or the news. Using examples from the media not only serves as a good segue into a conversation about sex, it also takes the focus off your teen. Amy Cody, Manager of Parent Education at Planned Parenthood League of Massachusetts, makes the point that "Talking about a sexual issue in reference to a movie makes a discussion less confrontational. It's not: What are you doing? What are your friends doing? But it still gives you some insight about what your kids are thinking." It also allows you to say your piece about a sexual issue without teens feeling like you're lecturing them specifically.

Keep It General

Even if you aren't talking about a sexual issue with regard to the media, it's best to keep your statements general, as opposed to focused on your teen. Saying something along the lines of "I think you're too young to have sex; you're just not ready" might illicit a response like, "What makes you think I'm having sex?" or "Why do you treat me like a child?" Rephrasing your line to "I think people tend to be better prepared to have sex when they are older" keeps the sentiment, but doesn't directly attack your teen. Keeping the subject of the conversation to "boys," "girls," "teens," or "young adults" will keep your child off the defensive.

Make It a Conversation

During a conversation, two people are talking and listening to each other's responses. When you're talking with your kids about sex, it should be a conversation, not a lecture. Don't be so concentrated on what you want to say to them, that you forget to listen to how they are responding to you. Be what therapists call an "active listener." Encourage your teen to keep talking by prompting him or her with phrases like: "What exactly do you mean by that?" or "It sounds like what you're saying is . . . ." By really listening to your teen's thoughts and concerns, you'll have a better sense of what topics need to continue to be explained, and which sexual issues your child may be struggling with.

Don't Rush Your Answers

As a parent, I'm sure there is a part of you that wants to be able to answer all of your kids' questions right away. But there will be some things that you won't feel prepared to talk about. Maybe your child has asked you a medical question and you're not sure of the answer. Or maybe it's a moral question and you're not sure how you feel about the issue. Either way, instead of forcing out an incomplete or knee-jerk answer, it's fine to take a time-out and come back to the topic later. Tell your child, "I'm not really sure. Let me get back to you about that." But do keep good on your promise, and return to the issue, even if you can't give an easy answer.

Know They're Listening

Just because your kids may not look enthralled by your thoughts about sex doesn't mean your insights are falling on deaf ears. Teens are listening; they might just act like they aren't because they feel awkward or don't know what to say in response. Think about it, I bet you remember everything your parents did (and didn't) say to you about sex . . . even though you probably acted pretty indifferent at the time.

Should Fathers Talk to Sons and Mothers to Daughters?

For kids who grow up in families with two different-sex parents, ideally both will take an active role in educating each one of their children. When possible, I do think that genital-related questions and more nitty-gritty sexual details may be most easily discussed with the same-sex parent. Most girls are probably more comfortable talking with their mothers about types of contraception, whether or not they have a yeast infection, or any other issue that's vagina specific. Likewise, boys are probably most comfortable talking with their fathers about how to use a condom, any concerns they have about their penises, or any graphic sexual topic. But since sexuality is a much broader issue than body concerns and the nuts and bolts of sexual intercourse, the opposite-sex parent can still add much to the discussion.

Especially when talking about romantic relationships, the opposite sex parent can be instrumental in helping to explain a guy's or girl's perspective. A father may be more likely to convince his daughter that a decent guy won't pressure her into sex, and a mother might be better able to help her son after a tough break up. Both parents should certainly be able to give their children insight about when sex is appropriate, how to treat a sexual partner, and how to demand to be treated in return. In general, two heads are better than one, and your child can likely benefit from two perspectives on any sexual issue that may arise.

Not all families have two different-sex parents that can or will talk about sex with their children—and that's okay too. Much more important than your biological sex is how good of a communicator you are and how much trust you can build with your teen. If you are a single mom with two sons, or a family of two dads and one daughter, you can still talk with your children about every issue necessary. It may mean that you have to go out of your comfort zone a little bit more, but you can still be just as effective a resource for your children. I look at it like this: many women prefer to have female gynecologists, but male gynecologists are just as capable of giving a pelvic exam. Though some matters may be more difficult to discuss with a different-sex child, what's most important is that you maintain an open and honest line of communication.

When in doubt, just say *something*. It may not have the best opening line, happen at the greatest time, or be the most articulate speech you've ever given, but who cares? The most important thing is to get the conversation flowing, and to get it flowing early. Possibly, earlier than you think. . . .

Chapter Three SEXUALITY AND RELATIONSHIP TOPICS FOR TWEENS

My mom's brother was gay, so when I came out to her as bisexual I thought that she of all people wouldn't have a problem with it. I told her one day when I was sixteen, and she got this look of horror and just said, "Really? . . . Oh." Over the next few years we had a few big fights about it, and although they always ended with "I love you" and "I'll love whoever you love," the way she acted told a different story. Overall we have a good relationship, but her inability to understand my sexual orientation has been a catalyst for all of my problems with her today.

—Laura, age twenty

Oh, eighth grade. It was the year Sean and Anna got caught making out in the woods and "Damn, it's a sports bra" became everyone's favorite quote. That was the year I had a boyfriend/boy friend/whatever he was, who wanted to talk to me on the phone for hours every day, otherwise he said he was going to kill himself. It was also the year I became aware of calories, and half the girls in my class developed eating disorders.

When I talk to parents, they always want to know: when does it all start? When do I need to start talking with my kids about sex—like *sex* sex. My answer to that is this: it all starts in middle school; grades six, seven, and eight (and possibly even before). Sure, the majority of middle schoolers aren't necessarily having sex—though according to the Youth Risk Behavior Survey (2007) a good third do before they enter high school. But even middle schoolers who aren't having intercourse may be starting to have romantic relationships, developing feelings about their bodies, starting to form opinions about sexuality, and beginning to engage in sexual activities (that may or may not include intercourse). Although most people's sexual orientation isn't solidified until later in their teens or twenties, middle school is the time gay youth may start to realize they're different. It's also the time when kids start tossing around the term "gay" as an insult or colorful adjective.

Some middle schoolers may be too young to start talking to about the more physical aspects of sex (like what birth control method works best, or the nuances of how to properly use a condom). But they are certainly old enough to start hearing about broader issues that have to do with sexuality and healthy relationships. The whole point of talking with your kids about sexual issues is to start the conversations *before* they need to actually utilize the advice. Besides, "whatever your kids aren't ready to hear they'll filter out," says Katharine O'Connell White, an

OB-GYN at Baystate Medical Center. "You cannot give kids too much information."

This chapter is about some of the initial topics to start discussing with your kids: technology and the media, body image, relationships, sexual assault, sexual orientation, and oral sex. The topics at the beginning of this chapter (technology and the media, body image, and healthy relationships) are all topics you may want to start discussing with your kids even before middle school. The ones toward the end of the chapter are issues you may want to discuss a bit later (seventh and eighth grade), depending on your child's maturity.

A NOTE ABOUT THE TERM "HOOKING UP"

Many parents are curious about the term "hooking up." You've probably heard your kids use it, heard it on TV, and read about it in newspapers, but you may not be completely sure what it means. Generally, the term is used one of two ways. The first way simply means the same thing as "getting it on." It's a vague term for sexual activity ranging from making out to having sex. For example: "We were hooking up and my brother walked in." Or, "She answered her phone mid hookup." The other way it is used is to describe a relationship where two people engage in some type of sexual act on a regular basis but aren't boyfriend and girlfriend, and sometimes aren't even going on dates (usually a type of relationship that would happen in college). For example: "We were hooking up the whole time she was dating Kevin." Or, "He's not my boyfriend, I'm just hooking up with him."

Sex, Technology, and the Media

It used to be that television was "the great American babysitter," but now with newer technology—iPods, portable DVD players, and that thing they call the inter-web—your TV has outsourced some of its responsibilities. If your kids are like most, they spend a good amount of their day watching/listening/surfing something—possibly something you barely know how to use. According to a recent survey, around 10 percent of all media that children use has sexual content, almost 40 percent of the music they listen to has sexual lyrics (Brown 2005), and less than 1 percent of the sexual content in the media could be considered a portrayal of healthy sexual behavior (Hust et al. 2008). For better or for worse (and until the media starts portraying healthier messages just *worse*), Hollywood is educating your kids about sex and relationships.

As easy as it is to get upset about this and call it a day, I didn't bring it up just to add something else onto your plate of concerns. In truth, the media can only be as much of an influence as you let it. I'm not suggesting that you ban anything with possible sexual content from your house. After all, as strict as you may want to be in your own home, your children are going to be exposed to sexual content eventually. Your job isn't necessarily to limit what they are exposed to (although you may want to do that anyway), it is to teach your kids to be smarter media consumers.

Find out what messages are being sent to your kids and confront them. Remind your kids that everything they're looking at isn't reality; it's entertainment. When an emotionally unavailable, sex-hungry guy gets all the girls on television, tell your kids: "That's not the kind of guy that girls want in real life." When a movie shows two gorgeous teen actors having hot Hollywood sex, protest how unrealistic it is that they never stopped to use a condom and that neither one is freaking out about pregnancy or STDs. Sit down with your daughter as she's leafing through a magazine and tell her about all the airbrushing they do to pictures and how if you saw a model in real life she would look nothing like that. As painful as it may be, let your child listen to his or her favorite radio station in the car, just so that you can hear "the type of crap" they're calling music these days. When a really sexual song comes on, talk about the lyrics: "All these rappers talking about pussy this, and bling that. They're just selling a tough-guy image. In real life they probably just go home to a golden retriever and cuddle."

A concern related to sexualized media that seems to be increasingly on parents' minds (and the talk show circuit) is sex and technology: kids sending sexual text messages, or posting provocative pictures on Facebook. But to blame technology for this behavior is blaming a symptom of a greater disease; dirty text messages aren't sending themselves. Contrary to what some sensationalistic media would like for you to believe (remember the lecture you just gave your kid, "media is entertainment"), the solution here is pretty simple. And it has less to do with eliminating cell phone and Facebook use and more to do with talking with your kids about appropriate ways of communicating. There will always be some new form of something that kids can use to sexually exploit themselves. Your goal is to keep them from thinking that's a good idea in the first place.

Let your kids in on a very important aspect of technology: It leaves a trail. Text messages can be shown to anyone; anything posted online lives forever, and everyone—a parent, teacher, coach, or future boss—has access to the Internet. Secondly, talk with your kids about what it means to respect themselves sexually. Tell them they should only act sexual with people they actually want to have sex with, and they should only have sex within a respectful and caring context (more about this in Chapters 4, 8, and 9). Although it may seem like less of a big deal to send a dirty text than it is to say the same thing to a person's face, essentially if they texted it, they said it. Tell them that if something is too risqué to say or do in front of someone, it's too risqué to text, send, or post. If it's not something they would show a teacher, say on TV, or print on the front page of the newspaper, it should not be posted online or sent in a text message.

REAL-LIFE ADVICE

The Internet can be a pretty vague concept. Help your child understand just how far-reaching and permanent the Internet and other forms of technology are by explaining it in concrete terms: "You need to be careful about what you send to people's cell phones or post online. Maybe you think you're sending a raunchy text as a joke, but you won't be able to prove that when the message is being circulated around your whole school. If you upload a picture of yourself naked onto Facebook, someone can copy that picture and years from now when you're running for mayor, starting your own business, or becoming a well-known artist it can resurface and ruin your reputation. When you're applying for colleges, going out for a sports team, or trying to get a job, the very people you are trying to impress can go online and see anything embarrassing you have ever posted. If it's not something you would send or post in front of me, don't do it."

The media, technology, and any other negative influence that hurls itself at your kid is nothing that you can't swat down. But in order to combat these influences you have to constantly be alert, aware, and willing to start talking.

Technology Guidance and Restrictions

Jane Brown, PhD, studies the effects media and technology have on kids at the University of North Carolina at Chapel Hill. She recommends these ways parents can oversee their children's use of the technology:

- Have kids earn the right to privacy on their cell phones and computers.
- Block inappropriate websites from the family computer.
- Know who is on your children's buddy lists and who they're friends with on Facebook.
- Tell your kids that if they ever feel uncomfortable about how someone is talking to them online they should just not respond.

The Body Image Battle

If you're a woman, especially a young woman, the chances of always feeling good about your body are slim. Women love to hate their bodies, we bond over it—it's almost a rite of passage to becoming an adult: "My ass is huge," "My arms jiggle," "If I eat that it will go straight to my hips." I don't think young men necessarily feel that amazing about their bodies, but I do believe they're generally less obsessed with them, making body image more explicitly a health concern for young women. And all this body critiquing is a health concern because it affects women's self-esteem, which in turn affects their ability to make healthy decisions. Young women who have a negative view of their bodies are less likely to demand that a condom be used and more likely to have unprotected sex (Salazar 2004). Helping your children, especially your daughters, feel better about their bodies is important, not just for their overall mental health but for their sexual health as well.

Of course, trying to impart a positive body image to your kids can be an uphill battle. For everything you say that's positive, there are hundreds of advertisements, magazine articles, TV shows, and fashion photos to counteract it. Even news programs tend to obsess about celebrities' weights, what they eat, what they don't eat, how fat they got while pregnant, and how quickly they got back to their prebaby size. This is yet another reason why you have to talk with your kids about the images they see on TV and in print, and help them analyze the messages the media sends.

Although you can't control what your kids will hear in the outside world, you can control what they hear in your house. Do your part by refusing to join into the body-obsessed culture. Don't comment on celebrities' weight, your friends' weight, their friends' weight, or even your own weight in front of your kids. If you go on a diet, don't make it the center of household discussion—even if it's on the forefront of your mind. And never, under any circumstances, comment on your children's weight (unless, of course, it is a health concern and you need to speak with them and their doctor). Even comments that may seem innocent to you, like, "You have the cutest chubby knees," or "I didn't know you wore a size six," could be devastating and embarrassing for your teen. I knew a girl whose eating disorder was triggered by her aunt innocently commenting on her "chipmunk cheeks." As a friend of mine puts it: "There are two things I've learned: you never talk to a girl about her weight or her mustache."

Another way you can work to counteract negative body image is by reminding your kids that the most important thing is for their body to stay healthy. Our body is our vehicle to move around in the world; it allows us to play sports, walk around the mall, hike up a mountain, swim at the beach, and dance at a party. Some of the extremes people go to in order to look a certain way cause so much damage that their body doesn't function like it used to. And what is the point of having a body in the first place if it's one you can't move around in and use to do the things you love? I knew a girl who eventually overcame anorexia because she was a soccer fanatic and wanted to play soccer more than she wanted to be unhealthily thin. Make the connection for your children that the way they treat their bodies affects their ability to take part in their favorite activities. Encourage your children to eat well and exercise because that's an important part of being healthy (not because it's an important part of looking a certain way). And make sure they know that being really thin is not any healthier than being really fat.

Something else you can do to help improve your kids' body image is to put their concerns about how they look into perspective. What exactly are they thinking they will achieve by being thinner (assuming they're at a healthy weight currently)? Young women in particular seem to take out all of their unhappiness on their body. They mistakenly think if they were five pounds thinner or one size smaller, all of their problems would go away. But really, having a flatter stomach, smaller thighs, perfect arms, or whatever else they fantasize about isn't going to change that much about their life. It's not going to make Mr. Not Interested come around, earn them more friends, make them more confident, or give them a more positive outlook on life. If your daughter suddenly seems interested in becoming stick thin, ask her what her motivation is. Chances are, there is an issue with a much more direct solution than dieting.

Eating Disorders

When dieting becomes an obsession, it becomes an eating disorder. Eating disorders may not be directly linked to teen sexuality, but they're tied to overall mental health and self-esteem, which in turn affect the choices your child will make regarding sex.

I worry that some parents have this perception of eating disorders: "So she gets a little skinny for a bit, then gets over it." Many don't understand just how dangerous it is to a person's health, or the reality that one out of five people with anorexia die prematurely because of complications associated with their disorder (Renfrew Center 2002). Just to put that number in perspective, that's a higher mortality rate than childhood leukemia, which at face value seems much more menacing than an eating disorder (St. Jude 2009).

REAL-LIFE ADVICE
You may want to slip this in at a time when your teen is looking at a magazine, watching TV, or making a negative comment about his or her body. "The most important thing about your body is that it's healthy, not what it looks like. Getting really skinny or doing anything unhealthy to make your body look a certain way can make you sick, damage your bones, and damage your muscles. And then you won't be able to do any of the things you love. You know how bad you feel when you're really sick, just stuck in bed, can't do anything, and nothing's fun because you feel so terrible. When you do something to mess up your body and your health, that's what you feel like all the time. You have to eat to live, and you have to be healthy to have fun."

Although eating disorders can affect anyone, they are most common in women and typically begin in a girl's teen years.

The two most common eating disorders are anorexia, when someone simply does not eat, and bulimia, when someone eats a lot, then throws it up, exercises obsessively, or takes laxatives to get the food out of his or her system. Someone who is anorexic is very skinny, whereas someone who is bulimic can look completely healthy. I had a friend who was bulimic, and every time my parents saw her they'd comment, "She doesn't look too skinny; she looks healthy to me." Like many, they had a hard time understanding that although my friend looked fine on the outside—as do many bulimics—on the inside her organs were a mess.

In order to catch an eating disorder, pay attention to your teen's eating habits—especially if she seems too skinny, has recently lost a lot of weight, seems obsessed with exercising, or always seems to be disappearing into the bathroom after meals. Answer these questions if you think your daughter could be anorexic:

Has your daughter recently lost a lot of weight, and does she seem unhealthily skinny and look sickly or malnourished?

Does she eat breakfast? And do you actually see her eat something, not just grab something from the kitchen then go back to her room?

Does she eat dinner in front of you, or does she make up excuses to skip dinner, saying she ate somewhere else?

During lunch she's at school, so you may have no way of knowing if she actually ate or not. As a general rule, if she looks too skinny, don't necessarily trust that she's eating enough, even if she tells you she has been.

Bulimia can be harder to recognize because bulimics are often a healthy weight and can appear to eat fairly normally. Be aware of any signs that your children are eating unnatural amounts of food and/or going to extremes to get the food out of their bodies. Answer these questions if you think your child could be bulimic:

Is food disappearing from the pantry?

Have you found food stashed away in your child's room?

Does your child seem to be unable to stop eating once he or she starts?

Does your child go right to the bathroom after eating and stay there for a while?

Does the bathroom smell like vomit if you walk in right after your child?

Can you hear your child throwing up if you listen closely?

Is your child running the water to mask the noise?

Does the nail on your child's pointer finger appear to be eroded (from vomiting on it after sticking it down his or her throat)?

Have you found laxatives in your child's room or backpack?

Pay special attention to your child's attitude: does he or she seem obsessive about exercising or burning calories?

If you're concerned that your child may have an eating disorder, it's not doing any good to sit around and worry about it. Talk to a doctor, call the national eating disorders association's helpline (1-800-931-2237), or speak with a trusted friend who has dealt with a similar issue.

Relationships

The time to start talking with your kids about what makes a healthy relationship is before they ever start dating. Timing is everything. Starting the conversation about what makes a good partner when your fourteen year-old daughter pulls up on the back of Frank, the seventeen-year-old dropout's, motorcycle is too late. Telling her it's a bad idea to date older guys with no ambitions goes from an easy conversation to an attack against her first love. So please, protect your kids from the Franks of the world before it's an issue, and talk with them about what makes a healthy relationship.

Healthy Relationships

On a basic level, kids need to understand that a healthy relationship is one that includes trust, respect, understanding, kindness, and equality. In a healthy relationship, two people talk to each other in a respectful way, put in equal effort, and the relationship adds to their overall happiness.

It may be useful to explain this by using your children's friendships as an example. I'm sure they have close friends with whom they have a very equal and loving relationship, as well as friends with whom they've had past problems. Help them understand romantic relationships by saying, "When you start dating, your relationship should be like your friendship with X, you have a lot of fun together, you're nice to each other, you both make time for each other, and you know you can rely on one another. Don't get involved with someone like Y, who has done such and such to upset you." Giving your children a concrete example of a healthy relationship can help make vague terms like "respect," and "trust" more palpable.

Kids also need to know how to keep a relationship healthy. Judging from the many teens I speak with every year, it's clear that any type of romantic relationship they get involved in consumes a significant amount of their life. It's also clear that many aren't always sure if that relationship is consuming them in a good way or a bad way. From what I've seen, many teens need help finding a balance between having a relationship and spending time pursuing their personal hobbies, goals, and other friendships. Jane Key, the sexual violence services coordinator for the South Carolina Department of Health, believes kids need to know: "You don't have to do everything your girlfriend/boyfriend does. You need to have the freedom to pursue your individual interests, or you get so wrapped up in your partner you lose yourself." Being new to romantic relationships is both exciting and overwhelming. When your children do start dating it may be helpful to remind them that if the relationship goes sour, it will be their friends and hobbies that will help them through the breakup.

Age is another factor that comes into play in young people's relationships. A healthy relationship means one between two teens that are roughly the same age. As you might remember from your own high school experience, dating someone much older happens way more often to young women—since it takes quite the fourteen-year-old boy to catch the attention of a much older girl. But miracles do happen, and whether it's a boy or a girl who is dating someone older, the toll it takes on his or her sexual health is quite significant. Studies show that teens in a relationship with someone three or more years older are significantly more likely to have sex earlier, less likely to use contraception, and more likely to report the sex as unwanted (Darroch 1999).

TMI WARNING

While you may want to talk with your children about your past relationships and some things you learned from them, make sure you stay focused on the emotional side of the relationship, not the sexual side. There is no reason to share things like: "She wasn't very nice, and she never put in as much effort as I did, but I stayed in the relationship a while because we had such great sex," or "I dated someone much older than me and he kept talking about wanting blow jobs, but I wasn't at all ready to put my mouth on a penis."

As an adult, it's easy to forget that a three-year age gap could cause such a power imbalance, but for teens, three years is a big deal. It's the difference between a freshman in high school and a senior in high school. There are always exceptions, but given the amount of changing and maturing teens do every year, what an older teen could want with someone much younger is a bit suspect. It makes me wonder, first of all, why that teen can't find someone his own age, and second, if that teen may be looking for someone younger in order to have all the power in the relationship. Again, before "Frank" comes along, speak with your kids about why you think it's a good idea for them to date someone their own age. Some benefits I've always found: there's more to talk about because you're going through the same things, the power feels more equal, you probably know more about the person because you know some of the same people, and you know the person is mature enough to be dating someone of equal age.

Unhealthy Relationships

Hands down, the scariest thing about your child beginning to date is the chance that he or she might become involved in an abusive relationship. One in five teens in a relationship have been hit, slapped, or pushed by their partner and one in four teen girls has been verbally abused by her partner. But perhaps what's most confusing is that nearly four out of five girls who have been physically abused stay with that partner (Liz Claiborne, Inc. 2005). Looking at these statistics you may wonder how so many teens get involved with assholes, and why they're dumb enough to stick around. But it's not that simple.

The problem with abusive relationships is that they're often a cycle. When the abuser isn't being abusive he may be really amazing: smart, good looking, personable, sweet, and funny. Maybe 90 percent of the time the relationship is flawless, but it's the 10 percent of the time it's not that's the issue. Abuse cycles because after a partner has been abusive he will promise he'll ever do it again, show how sorry he is, be incredibly sweet, and for a while the relationship will go back to being perfect. And of course, the victim wants to believe he won't do it again because she's in love.

Although the majority of the time the abuser is a "he," teens need to know that both men and women can be abusive. Abuse can be physical and include punching, shoving, hitting, and choking, but it can also be more subtle and include behaviors teens may not initially recognize as abuse. Making threats, trying to intimidate someone, humiliating someone, constantly putting someone down by telling them they're stupid, ugly, or worthless, or trying to isolate them from friends and family are all behaviors that count as abuse. And those are also behaviors that a woman can just as easily do to a man. Abuse can be mental and emotional as well as physical, and teens should understand that any kind of abuse is just as wrong as hitting someone.

REAL LIFE ADVICE

Next time you're with your child and you see a couple arguing in the grocery store, go to a friend's house where the couple has an unhealthy relationship, or hear a news story about abuse on the radio, take the opportunity to start talking about healthy relationships. Tell your teen something like: "In a healthy relationship two people are kind to each other, respect each other, trust each other, and put in equal effort. I'm sure you know that when you start dating it's never okay for the person you're with to hit you or physically hurt you in any way. But it's also not okay for them to say mean things to you, try to control you, threaten you, try to force you to do something you're not comfortable with, or try to intimidate you by getting violent—even if you're in a fight. Although 95 percent of the time your girlfriend/boyfriend may be perfect, acting this way even 5 percent of the time is a problem. You know if you ever have any questions about the way someone is treating you, you can come to me and ask."

Sexual Assault

To help prevent your daughter from getting sexually assaulted you may tell her not to walk alone at night, not to talk to strangers, and to always keep the doors and windows locked. In general, not bad advice, but as far as sexual assaults are concerned, that advice is a bit irrelevant. In two out of three rapes, the victim knows her attacker: he is a friend, a partner, or even a relative—he isn't some stranger who jumped out from behind a dumpster (RAINN 2009). (And it's important to keep in mind that guys can be victims of sexual assault too.)

Date Rape

Much more common than stranger rape is date rape, when a girl voluntarily goes off alone with a guy she knows and trusts. Maybe it's even a guy she's initially interested in and willingly starts to make out with, but then he forces her to have sex. Both young men and young women should understand what the typical rape scenario looks like: two people who know each other—not a deranged man with a crowbar in a back alley.

Because so many teens don't fully understand that date rape counts as rape, many victims don't know that what happened to them was sexual assault. As a result, they think the incident was their fault. They blame themselves for initially giving off the wrong impression, making the decision to go off alone with someone, or not having better judgment. Then, thinking they caused it, they don't tell anyone about the attack, don't seek help, and many turn to unhealthy ways of coping.

According to the RAINN website (Rape, Abuse, and Incest National Network), rape is defined as "forced sexual intercourse, including vaginal, anal or oral penetration." It's important to know that the term "force" doesn't just include physical force, but encompasses psychological force such as verbal or physical threats. For example, if a girl's boyfriend gets her to have sex by saying, "let me do it or I'm going to break every piece of furniture in your room/tell everyone at school you're a whore/punch you in the stomach," that is rape. It doesn't matter that she didn't try to fight him off (many victims don't because they are too scared, or know realistically they're not strong enough). It also doesn't matter that the girl had sex with him willingly in the past, and might again in the future, or that he's technically her boyfriend. Teens need to understand that rape is *any* situation where sex is not a mutual decision.

SEXUAL ASSAULT IS A SERIOUS ISSUE
One out of every six women has been the victim of a completed or attempted rape.

One out of every thirty-three men has been the victim of an attempted or completed rape.

Forty percent of sexual assaults and rapes take place in the victim's home, 20 percent take place in the home of a friend, neighbor, or relative, and 8 percent take place in a parking garage.

Victims of sexual assault are twenty-six times more likely to abuse drugs.

Only 60 percent of rapes and sexual assaults are reported to the police.

Only 6 percent of rapists will ever spend a day in jail.

All statistics taken from the RAINN website: *www.rainn.org*

Help your children develop a firm grasp on date rape, but also help them understand the importance of both setting and respecting sexual boundaries. Encourage your daughters to speak up for themselves in sexual situations. If they ever feel uncomfortable while hooking up with someone, tell them to say something like "no," "stop," or "I don't want this to go any further." If they are ever in a situation where a guy is trying to pressure them into sex, tell them to clearly state: "I do not want to have sex with you, and if you make me, it is rape." In some situations, a guy (especially if he is a boyfriend) may not be aware that what he's doing is starting to cross the line. If he is explicitly told, he may be more likely to back off. That being said, a guy should never have to be reminded not to rape his girlfriend, and a rape isn't a girl's fault if she doesn't verbalize "what you're doing to me is rape."

REAL-LIFE ADVICE

Bring this up if you've recently seen a movie with a rape scene, if there's a news story about a rape case, or if you hear your child talking about rape. If none of those opportunities present themselves, just start talking: "Usually, rapes happen between two people who know each other—two people on a date, two people who go off alone at a party, or even two people in a relationship. Whenever someone makes clear they don't want a hookup to go any further, their partner needs to stop. It's not okay for anyone, even a boyfriend, to try to force a girl into sex. It's even wrong if he's forcing her by making verbal threats. Sex always needs to be a mutual decision. And if someone is really drunk or sleeping, it's not."

Teach your sons to always respect any sexual boundaries a girl has set. But beyond that, teach him to always check in with his partner. Encourage him to ask, "Is this okay," "are you still all right," or "do you want me to stop?" Tell him to be on the lookout for signs that a girl is uncomfortable, and if he notices any to say something. Whenever there is a doubt as to whether sexual contact is wanted or not, the responsible thing to do is to stop and ask.

Sexual Orientation

Sexual orientation: gay or not, I'd say it's something everyone pauses to think about, at least once or twice. Sexual orientation is confusing for many teens because the majority of people aren't actually 100 percent gay or 100 percent straight. So every now and then they might have thoughts, feelings, and fantasies that contradict their sexual "label." The famous sexologist Alfred Kinsey theorized that sexuality is a continuum, with complete heterosexuality on one side, and complete homosexuality on the other. After years of research, he concluded that the majority of people fall somewhere along that line, but not exactly at one end or the other.

Because everyone's sexuality is in essence a shade of gray, many teens struggle when trying to categorize their sexual preference as one or the other: "I usually like girls but I'm really enjoying being around this guy—am I gay or am I straight?" Many don't know that just because they may have a sexual thought about someone of the same sex it doesn't necessarily mean they're gay. Similarly, just because they may have had sexual experiences with someone of the opposite sex, that doesn't necessarily make them straight. Talk with your kids about sexual orientation, and explain that one's sexual preference is determined by who they're attracted to the *majority* of the time. That may not always be who they've had sex with in the past, who they'll have sex with in the future, or who they rarely have crushes on. Young people who do eventually identify as homosexual often start to suspect they may be gay in their teens. As their friends are starting to get preoccupied with the opposite sex, gay teens don't really get what the fuss is about. As a result, they might feel confused, left out, and different from those around them—feelings that many teens experience anyway, but are often amplified for those who are gay. That distress can then lead to depression and self-destructive behaviors.

One study found that lesbian and bisexual teens are actually more likely to have had vaginal intercourse than heterosexual teens. And when gay and bi youth did have sex, they were also less likely to use protection (Saewyc et al. 1999). Although on the one hand it doesn't make sense that girls who like other girls would be having sex with boys, it also doesn't take a rocket scientist to guess what's going through their heads when they do: maybe if I have straight sex it will prevent me from being gay? Maybe if I have straight sex no one will suspect I am gay? Maybe if I have straight sex I'll feel normal like everyone else? As a parent, you can help your children process their sexual identity in a way that can help them avoid depression and dangerous sexual choices. You can help them understand that their sexuality is determined by what they feel and who they're attracted to, not who they have sex with.

Of course, it goes without saying that helping your children have healthy thoughts about sexual preference means having a tolerant and understanding view yourself.

Recently I asked a lesbian friend of mine what parents should know about sexual orientation. She said this: "I wish they would understand that it's not a choice. People don't mentally decide to be gay; they are physically attracted to people of the same sex. I explain it this way: if I were walking in the woods and there were two paths, one that was perfectly cleared and another that was overgrown with weeds, rocks, and branches, I wouldn't *choose* to walk down the more difficult path. Being a lesbian is more challenging than being straight; it's not something I chose to be for fun. I'm not trying to be attracted to other women, I just am."

REAL-LIFE ADVICE

Bring this up next time you hear your teen mention the word "gay," see a story about homosexual rights, or see a TV show with a gay character. You can also open up the topic with a question like: "Do people at your school use the term 'gay' as an insult?" "Do any kids in your class have two moms?" or "are there any openly gay people at your school?" Then tell your teens this: "Many people believe that no one is 100 percent gay, or 100 percent straight, but that everyone's sexuality falls somewhere between the two extremes. Your sexual orientation is really about who you're attracted to the majority of the time. It's not necessarily dependant on who you have sex with. If you're attracted to (boys/girls), it's not going to make you straight by sleeping with a lot of (girls/boys). It's all about what you feel, not necessarily what you do. And I hope you know that I love you no matter what, and if you figured out you were gay, you could always tell me and I'd be here to help you with that."

Oral Sex

A few years back there was a great deal of hubbub about middle schoolers having oral sex parties, having oral sex in casual relationships, and just generally going down on people at inappropriate times. Although for a while it seemed like a blowjob was becoming the latest bar mitzvah gift, no studies show that casual oral sex is actually a widespread middle school norm.

What research has supported, however, is the fact that some teens that aren't having intercourse are having oral sex (about a third to be exact). When asked why a teen has engaged in oral sex but not intercourse, these are some of the common answers they gave: because of their religion/morals, to avoid pregnancy, to avoid STDs, because they haven't met the right partner, and because it wasn't the right time (The National Campaign to Prevent Teen and Unplanned Pregnancy 2005). Quite simply, oral sex doesn't matter to teens as much as intercourse. The red flags this information raises are (1) that teens may not know they can get STDs from oral sex, and (2) that some don't see oral sex as a big deal (it's okay with God, they can do it with Mr. or Ms. Wrong, and they don't have to be as emotionally prepared).

The emphasis that widespread abstinence-only sex education has placed on virginity has backfired in that it's inadvertently encouraged sex acts other than penis-in-vagina intercourse. I went to a conservative southern high school where a lot of the girls were told they should save themselves for marriage. Wanting to stay true to their religion, they only had anal sex with their boyfriends, and walked around heads held high because they were still virgins. The cultural obsession with virginity has lead to some absurd choices. Because vaginal intercourse is what most people mean by "having sex" (as far as the term "virgin" is concerned), many teens believe that other acts don't count.

Teens need to know that whether it affects their status as a virgin or not, all sex acts matter. Although some STDs are probably less likely to be transmitted through oral sex, it's not a completely "safe" activity. Anal sex is actually riskier than vaginal sex as far as STDs are concerned. But all infections aside, everything teens go through to decide if they're ready for intercourse should apply to other sex acts as well. Feeling used, regretful, or vulnerable is not unique to vaginal sex. Teens should be told that all of the bad emotions someone might experience from having intercourse in the wrong situation can be experienced from having *any* type of sex in the wrong situation. Sex is sex is sex. And with all sex acts, teens need to make sure they're truly ready, they're doing it with a caring and supportive partner, and it's something they're doing for the right reasons.

REAL-LIFE ADVICE

Ask your teens how they would describe a virgin. If they say they don't know, prompt them with scenarios: "Is someone who has had oral sex a virgin? What about anal sex? What about touched someone else's penis/vagina?" Then, launch into this advice: "Even though you can engage in some sex acts and still technically be considered a virgin, all types of sex matter. Even if it can't make a girl pregnant, oral sex and anal sex can still spread STDs. And actually, you're more likely to get an STD through anal sex than you are from vaginal sex. Always choose carefully when you want to have sex and who you want to have sex with, and that goes for oral sex too."

TOPICS FOR TWEENS CHEAT SHEET

Here's a summary of the topics covered in this chapter, the major issues to discuss with your kids, and the important things to tell them:

1. Use the sexual content in the media to your advantage by having it serve as a jumping off point for conversations about sex. Remind your kids that what they see/hear is entertainment, not reality. Pay attention to what they're watching, reading, and listening to, and talk with them about the messages they're getting from the material.
2. Make sure your children know that respecting themselves carries over to cell phones, the Internet, and any other device. A good rule of thumb is to never send a text message you wouldn't say to someone's face, or a picture of something you'd be embarrassed to show them in person.
3. Everyone has things they don't love about their body, and that's okay. The most important thing about someone's body is that it is healthy. If it's not healthy, they can't continue to do all of the activities they love.
4. In a healthy relationship there is trust, respect, kindness, understanding, and equality, and both people keep their own separate lives and interests. For teens, the best relationships are those between two people of roughly the same age.
5. Abusive relationships can happen to anyone, and the abuse often happens in a cycle, interspersed with great times in the relationship. Abuse can be mental and emotional as well as physical.
6. Date rape (where the victim and attacker know each other) is much more common than stranger rape. Any-

time one person says no and is then physically or verbally forced into sex, it is rape.

7. Sexual orientation is a continuum, with gay on one end and straight on the other. Most people fall at some point on that line, but not at one end or the other. A person's sexual orientation is based on how they feel, not necessarily what they do.
8. Oral sex matters. Even though a person can have oral sex and still technically be a virgin, it carries many of the same risks and repercussions as sexual intercourse. A person needs to think carefully before he or she engages in oral sex.

Chapter Four WHEN IS SEX OKAY?

> ***Sex itself isn't good or bad, it has the potential to be either. But more than anything it's a powerful act.***
>
> ***—Charlie Buckholtz, rabbi and coauthor of*** **In Heaven Everything Is Fine: The Unsolved Life of Peter Ivers and the Lost History of New Wave Theatre**

As a teen, there was nothing more annoying or cliché than one of my parents' friends commenting on how big I'd gotten. I promised myself I'd never be one of those annoying old people who said things like, "I can't believe how much you've grown." Then, this summer, I ran into a girl I used to babysit for when she was two. She had boobs. Without being able to stop it, all I could say was, "You're so grown up," which was code for, "Crap, *I'm* a grown-up!" I didn't feel that much different from the way I felt when I was her babysitter, but this girl whose diapers I changed now had breasts and a boyfriend. Whether I wanted to be aware of it or not, many years had passed, and I was getting older.

I can only imagine that the thought of your child becoming sexually active must stir up similar feelings: How did I get so old? A friend of mine has a teenage niece who just started taking oral contraception because she's sexually active. My friend says that when she looks at her niece, all she can see is birth control pills. She can't believe that her brother's little kid is becoming a young adult—and having sex—when it seems like just yesterday she was playing with dolls.

One day, your child too will become sexually active, and though it may make you feel old, it's not the worst thing in the world. Culturally there seems to be the notion that parents should do everything in their power to make sure their kids (especially their daughters) don't have sex. And in trying to do that, some parents present sex as a montage of worst-case scenarios of irresponsible sexual choices. Reverend David O'Leary, the university chaplain at Tufts, finds irony in how many people go about trying to prevent teens from having sex: "They say sex is the filthiest and most disgusting thing in the world . . . which is why you save it for marriage. That's a pretty backwards and contradictory message if you ask me."

If you try to prevent your kids from having sex by telling them sex is inevitably upsetting, what happens when they do eventually have sex? But more importantly, if your kids expect sex to be horrible, how will they be able to recognize when they're having sex in the wrong situation with the wrong partner (isn't sex *supposed* to be bad)? Yes, sex *can* be painful, it can make people feel used, and lead to a whole range of emotions you never want your kids to feel. But it's not the physical act of sex that's responsible for those consequences; it's sex in the wrong situation.

Sex is a normal and healthy part of human development. As a parent, your job isn't to prevent sex from ever happening, it's to make sure it happens under the right circumstances. But what are the right circumstances? Marriage? A certain age? A declared monogamous relationship? There are no clear-cut answers to that question, and everyone's point of view is going to be different. This chapter will help you explore your ideas about when sex is okay. I hope it encourages you to look past concrete labels, ages, and restrictions, and instead helps you focus on the characteristics of a respectful relationship and a mature teen. I also hope it teaches you how to express your values but at the same time remain a resource for your child when the two of you can't see eye to eye.

You Can Have Sex When You're Married

Perhaps the easiest go-to-answer (and in some circles the *only* answer) for when sex is okay is: "when you're married." But like many easy answers, simple solutions to complex questions don't always cut it. Now that the average age of marriage is twenty-seven, saving sex for one's wedding night just isn't realistic. Honestly, can we ask adults to remain virgins through the better part of their twenties and expect them to comply? And even if they would, you have to wonder, is waiting for marriage even a good idea?

Any relationship therapist would tell you that sex is a very important part of marriage. Deciding to marry someone without ever knowing what the sex is like isn't a risk most people want to take. But beyond that, many feel that experiencing sex and intimate relationships with a few different people may help them to be better prepared to ultimately pick a mate. Sex before marriage isn't only the most realistic option; for many, it may also be the best.

As a parent, it's okay to approve of your children getting some sexual experience before they settle down with a life partner—and it's not just radicals who think this way. My mother is friends with a woman living in the deep South who is part of a traditional religious community. According to her friend's account, when the issue of premarital sex came up in her women's group, even though all of the women considered themselves to be devout Christians, not one of them wanted their children to wait until marriage to have sex. They all wanted their kids to experience sex with at least a few different people before they decided on a spouse. This, of course, was not a view they felt comfortable expressing publicly. But privately, they saw little value in the "abstinence until marriage" mentality.

I understand that some of you will never want to—or be able to—condone premarital sex. But there is a difference between saying sex before marriage is okay and educating your kids about sex. You can tell your kids you believe sex is only appropriate within a marriage, and that is the choice you want them to make. You can then tell them that just in case they don't make that choice, you want to talk with them about sexual health and sexual decision making.

Think of it this way: you tell your kids to always wear their seat belts. You say this not because you condone unsafe driving, or because you are encouraging them to crash into another car. You tell them to wear their seat belts *just in case* an accident happens. Teaching your kids about safer sex, and how to make good sexual decisions is information they can use *if* they decide to have sex. It is not the same as telling them they *should* have sex or that you think premarital sex is okay.

TMI WARNING

When helping your teen think about when sex is okay, don't share stories about losing your virginity, your early sexual experiences, or your "experiments" in college. Your teens will not find it enlightening; they will find it frightening.

Even university chaplain David O'Leary believes there has to be a middle ground between religious values and your child's sexual health needs. His concern is "if all you're telling your kids about sex is 'no,' where do they get information if they decide to become sexually active?" He suggests that religious parents can start conversations about sex by "leading with their own love, and saying they don't want their child to experience pain, or get hurt. Then discussions of protection and STDs can come from there." Explaining to your kids that you're giving them information because their health and well-being is your first priority will help to clarify that while you don't approve of them having sex, your primary concern is always their safety.

You Can Have Sex When You're in College or Otherwise out of My House

The difference between a freshman in college and a senior in high school is about three months. Anyone who wasn't emotionally or physically prepared to have sex in high school certainly isn't going to be magically ready the instant he or she sets foot on a college campus. But for some reason, many see high school as a time when sex is inappropriate and focus on college as a place where sex is okay.

A friend of mine tells a story about his freshman year in college: "There was this one girl on campus my friends and I referred to as 'the girl who has sex.' We were all convinced this girl would have sex with you right away if you dated her. She was the chick to go to if you wanted to get some. We later found out she was actually a lesbian and exclusively dated women."

To me, the moral of his story is that even college students aren't necessarily that sexually knowledgeable. The other moral is that just because someone is in college doesn't mean they're mature enough to be a good sexual partner. "The girl who has sex?" That'll be enough, buddy, go back to your video games.

Setting a specific age or circumstance for when sex is okay is a bad idea. The last thing you want is to give your teen an easy out when making sexual decisions: "I'm old enough to have sex, so I guess I'll go for it." The decision to become sexually active should come from a variety of factors, not a mentality of "I'm in college now; look what I can do!"

I knew many girls who had sex for the first time a few months into freshman year with guys they hardly knew. They assumed that since they were old enough to have sex, the situation they had sex in didn't matter. Of course, the situation did matter, and for the most part, their experiences weren't good ones. Since graduating, I have since spoken to many—guys and girls—who became sexually active only because they thought they were old enough, not because they were truly ready, or actually desired to have sex.

The message that "sex is okay in college," only adds to the pressure many teens feel to have sex when they reach campus. It's understandable how telling your kids they "can" have sex in college could morph into the idea they "should" have sex. Because sex in college is presented as acceptable, commonplace, and even inevitable, many students feel like they can't stay a virgin once they enter college, or that they can't say no to sex within a college relationship. The last thing you want to do is support those misconceptions.

Telling your kids they can have sex when they're in college or when they reach a certain age is just too arbitrary of a guideline. While it's okay to encourage your kids to wait until they are older because they might be better equipped to deal with the responsibilities that come along with sex, leave an exact age out of it.

You Can Have Sex Within a Serious Relationship or Once You're in Love

The baby-making process is stereotypically explained to kids with the legendary opening line, "When two people love each other very much . . . ." Years later, when parents are explaining to their kids when sex is appropriate, they often recycle that sentiment, or modify it to "when you're in a serious monogamous relationship." But just like "When you're in college," isn't a complete enough answer, "When you have a serious boyfriend or girlfriend," or "When you're in love," doesn't cut it either.

The first problem with using a type of relationship to determine when sex is appropriate is the fact that as an adult, your definitions are likely fairly different from your teens'. What you consider to be serious and what they consider to be serious are probably two very different scenarios. When I was fifteen, I thought I was in a majorly committed relationship because my boyfriend and I had been a couple for three months, saw a movie together every weekend, and talked on the phone every night. As intense as I considered my feelings to be then, looking back on it as an adult, I see it as little more than a high school crush.

At the time, however, had my parents tried to convince me my feelings weren't significant—or that the relationship wasn't serious—all hell would have broken loose. And if they tried to tell me I may not have actually been in love with the guy I dated later on in high school, I probably would have threatened to run away. One of the quickest ways to lose credibility with a teen is to imply their feelings don't count. And if you tell your teen sex is okay within a "serious relationship," it's likely that one day you'll have to backpedal and explain that their fifteen-year-old puppy love isn't exactly what you meant by serious. So rather than entering a heated debate about what constitutes a "real" relationship, "strong feelings," or "true love," it's best to leave vague labels out of your sex talk all together.

When it comes down to it, the nature of a relationship is much more important than the label attached to it. Anyone can call someone a boyfriend or girlfriend, and anyone can say, "I love you." But those labels are just words—that may or may not be describing a mature loving relationship.

It's always important to think about how your messages could be misinterpreted or how your words might come back to bite you. Again, it's understandable how a teen might make the jump from "Sex is okay within a serious relationship," to "Once you're in a serious relationship you can/should have sex." You never want to plant the seed that sex is a requirement of a certain relationship. It's very possible that a teen may start dating or even fall in love much before he or she is ready to have sex. For that reason, the decision to have sex should not be presented as synonymous with the feeling of being in love or the label of having a boyfriend or girlfriend.

So What Advice *Can* You Give?

I'm terrified of flying, and every time I meet a pilot I ask him to explain to me why planes are actually a safe way to travel. One pilot put it to me this way: for a plane to crash, it's not just one thing that has to go wrong—many things have to malfunction all at once.

I look at sex the same way (though, instead of lots of things needing to go wrong, it's lots of things that need to go right). For sex to be a good idea, it can't just be for one reason: "I'm in college" or "we love each other." For sex to be a good idea, many different internal and external factors have to fall into place. There isn't one easy answer to the question "When is sex okay?" because the answer can't be based on absolute terms or debatable definitions.

When describing a relationship where sex might be appropriate, instead of resorting to labels, consider discussing the following guidelines with your children. And let them know that these guidelines should go for every person they have sex with, not just the first.

- **A relationship that includes mutual respect**. Your teens should know that they shouldn't be having sex with someone who doesn't respect them (or someone they don't respect). Explain that respect means their partner values them, feels lucky to be with them, looks out for their interests and concerns, and pays attention to their needs and what makes them happy. A person who doesn't make time, put forth effort, or concern themselves with their partner's well-being isn't being respectful.
- **A relationship where they are comfortable**. A relationship is only ready for sex when both people feel truly comfortable. That means your teens should be able to freely share their thoughts, fears, and concerns with their

partner, and feel secure enough to get angry or upset if they have to.

- **A relationship based on trust.** Your teens should never consider having sex in a relationship without trust. And I mean trust in every sense of the word. Trust that their partner wants to do it for the right reasons, that they'll be there the next day, that they'll call when they say they will, that they won't go around spreading rumors, and that they'll be honest about their sexual history. Teens also need to trust themselves within the relationship and know that they want to have sex for the right reasons too.

REAL-LIFE ADVICE

Explain the type of relationship when sex is appropriate to your teen like this: "Before you have sex you should make sure the relationship you're in includes respect, comfort, and trust. People who respect you won't pressure you into having sex because they'll only want you to do it if you really want to. If you feel truly comfortable with someone, you can share all your thoughts, fears, or concerns, and you feel secure enough in the relationship that you can get angry or upset. Before you have sex you have to trust that your partner wants to do it for the right reasons, that he/she will be there for you the next day, and that down the road he/she will help you deal with any possible consequences, like STDs or an unplanned pregnancy. And perhaps most of all, you need to trust yourself—that you're not having sex only because your partner wants to, to impress your friends, or because you're expecting the relationship to get better by doing it—because it won't."

As important as it is for a teen to have sex in the right type of romantic relationship, it's equally as important that a teen has sex only once he or she feels personally ready as well. A relationship might be very loving and mature, but someone who isn't ready to have sex isn't ready to have sex, period, end of story. When talking to your child about what it means to be ready for sex on a personal level, consider discussing the following:

- **Emotional and Spiritual Readiness.** In order for sex to be a good idea, teens must be both emotionally and spiritually ready. If having sex in a certain situation contradicts their religious or moral values, they need to be at peace with that contradiction and believe sex is the right choice anyway. As far as emotions are concerned, they need to feel stable enough to handle any negative repercussions that could come as a result of having sex, as well as the added stress of worrying about STDs and pregnancy.
- **Physically Readiness**. During sexual intercourse a guy's penis goes inside a girl's vagina. If that idea still makes your daughter feel uncomfortable, or your son still says "gross" when you say the word "vagina," your kids aren't physically ready to have sex. The other component to being physically ready is being aware of the risks involved, and being prepared with contraception and condoms to help protect against an unplanned pregnancy and STDs.
- **Internal Desire.** Your teens will not be happy they had sex unless they did it for themselves. They need to have sex because *they* want to, not because they're feeling pressure from an outside source like a partner, friend, or the pressure to "lose it before a certain age."

REAL-LIFE ADVICE

Explain to your teen the signs that he or she is personally prepared to have sex. Tell your teen: "Before you have sex you have to be sure that you're doing it in a situation that lines up with your values. You also have to be sure that you're prepared emotionally for the possibility of feeling vulnerable and for the added stress and responsibility of being sexually active. On a physical level, you can't be grossed out by your partner's genitals or your own. And you should be physically prepared for sex with condoms and contraception. Most of all, you need to make sure that you want to have sex because *you* want to have sex, not because your partner wants to, you want to tell your friends you did, or you're tired of being a virgin."

It probably feels scary to give your kids open-ended advice and relationship concepts to think about instead of solid rules about when sex is acceptable. But you really can't give rules when it comes to sex, because you have no way of enforcing them. You are much better off getting your children to think critically about their sexual decisions. If they are really conscious about the choices they are making, they won't feel ready to have sex until they're in their late teens/early twenties and in a serious relationship anyway. But having them reach that conclusion on their own is much more powerful than you telling them what to do.

THE "WHAT IF" GAME

Need something to talk to your hubby about before bedtime? Need something else to debate with your ex? Want to put your nanny on the spot? Play this game with your spouse, the other parent of your child, anyone else prominent in your child's life.

What would you do if . . .

(Insert child's name here) told you he/she was having sex?

(Child's name) said he/she was thinking about having sex?

You found condoms or birth control pills in (child's name)'s backpack?

(Child's name) came to you upset because he/she had unprotected sex?

(Child's name) asked you to take him/her to the store to buy condoms or the doctor to get birth control?

Ultimately, the only way to control your children's behavior when it comes to sex is by influencing the way they think. When they're alone with their crush late one night at a party they snuck out to, you can't tell them what they can and cannot do because you won't be there. What will be there, however, are the values you instill in them. And in the end, those alone will guide their sexual choices.

What If They Go Against Your Guidance and Do It Anyway?

There's a possibility that one day, before you're ready to hear it, your child is going to tell you he or she is sexually active, is thinking about becoming sexually active, or made a bad sexual decision and needs your support. Should any of these occur, it's important to have thought about your response beforehand. That way, you avoid a heat-of-the-moment reaction: "You had sex? You're grounded! Forever!"

If your child tells you he or she went against your guidance, is planning to go against your guidance, or made an unwise sexual decision, chances are your first reaction may be anger and frustration. Even though it may be difficult, I'd encourage you not to get angry. I think it's always better to know what your child is doing (or thinking about doing) rather than being kept in the dark. If he or she opens up to you about sex and you just get angry, I doubt you'll be consulted again. And if your own children can't come to you, where do they go if they need help getting contraception or engaging in safer sex? As a general rule, you can applaud teens for being honest—by verbally thanking them and not reacting in anger—while at the same time clearly stating you don't approve of such behavior. The following are four different scenarios of things your teen might reveal to you, and a suggestion of how to react.

1. **Situation: Your teen says he or she is sexually active, seems happy with that decision, and plans on continuing to have sex. You, however, think he or she is too young or not in a relationship where sex is appropriate.** At this point, what's done is done. Getting angry isn't going to change what has happened or change your child's mind. You can always ground your child, but that

will only temporarily stop him or her from being able to have sex.

Your best bet is to say your first concern is that he or she is having sex safely. After making that clear, you might want to get in a *discussion* (note, I did not say lecture) about why your teen feels ready for sex, and why you feel he or she is not. Explain that you are only questioning the decision to have sex because you care and want to help him or her make the best choices.

2. **Situation: Your teen says he or she had sex in a bad situation, or unsafely, and is coming to you upset and concerned.** When teens come to their parents upset and concerned, they know they messed up. They aren't coming for a lecture about bad choices, or to get yelled at for making a stupid decision (and neither of these reactions is likely to help them at the time or in the long run). Your first concern should be dealing with the immediate problem: possibly by buying a pregnancy test, taking him or her to the doctor to get tested for STDs, or perhaps just being a shoulder to cry on. Your second order of business should be talking with your teen about why he or she made such a choice and what will make it easier to make a better choice in the future. Lastly, reinforce the idea that you will always be there for your child, no matter what, and that he or she can always come to you for support.

3. **Situation: Your teen tells you he or she is thinking about having sex, and you think it's a bad idea.** The fact that your child feels comfortable enough to talk

to you about a big decision *before* making it is a really good sign. Even if you think becoming sexually active is a horrible idea for your child, show him or her the same maturity you have been shown. Calmly and rationally discuss all of the personal and relationship components you believe must be in place before becoming sexually active. Say that you worry about him or her having to deal with some of the emotional issues that sex can bring up and that you think it's a better idea to wait a bit longer and spend some more time thinking about it and feeling out the relationship he or she is in. Throughout the whole conversation, keep reminding your teen you have his or her best interests in mind and are just trying to help him or her reach a decision that will be the best in the long run.

4. **Situation: You find birth control pills or condoms hidden in your child's belongings.** This scenario is tricky because the presence of contraception doesn't necessarily mean your child is sexually active—although, it's probably a sign it's at least a possibility. It's also tricky because on the one hand, it's good that he or she is being prepared, but on the other, you are not being kept in the loop. Before you do anything, you have to ask yourself: "Do I have the type of relationship where I'd expect to be told when my kid starts having sex?" and "Do I even want my teen to tell me?" Depending on your answers to those questions, you can decide if you want to tell your child explicitly about what you found. But either way, talk to your child again (or for the first time) about your values of when sex is appropriate, and reinforce the importance of having safer sex (just because condoms are there doesn't

> necessarily mean they will be used). Also tell your teen that if he or she is thinking about having sex, you want to do everything in your power to help make sure it is safe. Then reiterate that you're always happy to talk about any concerns he or she may have.

No matter what the situation, a good rule of thumb for your reaction should be safety first. Tattoo it into your skull, and anytime you're faced with a difficult or upsetting confrontation, pause to ask yourself: "How can I react in a way that is most likely to help my child make safe choices when it comes to sex?" Father David O'Leary advises, "You want your children to know that even if bad things happen, they can always come back to their parents. When parents just get angry over kids' bad sexual choices, where do they go then for guidance and information? Some important lessons can be learned from times when one fails. Parents can help kids process their failures, and learn from their mistakes."

Communicating Sexual Values: A Recap

Old habits die hard. It may be challenging to get used to the idea of telling your teen to have sex in a relationship with respect, trust, comfort, and security as opposed to "marriage," "love," or "college." To help get you in the habit, here are some suggested alternatives for some old go-tos.

Instead of telling your kids: "You can't have sex until you're married, no ifs, ands, or buts about it."

Try saying: "I believe sex is only appropriate within a marriage, and I would like you to wait until you're married to have sex. But, if you do decide to have sex before you get married, I want you to be safe about it." Then teach them about condoms and other forms of contraception.

Instead of telling your kids: "As long as you're living in my house, you live by my rules, and you're not having sex. When you get to college you can do whatever you want."

Try saying: "You shouldn't have sex until you feel completely emotionally, physically, and spiritually ready, and feel mature enough to be able to deal with the possible consequences. If you're honest with yourself, that probably won't be until you're older."

Instead of telling your kids: "Only have sex with a boyfriend/girlfriend who says, 'I love you.'"

Try saying: "Sex will only be enjoyable in a relationship where there is mutual trust and emotional security—when you know the person you had sex with will be there for you the next day, and in return, you know you'll be there for that person."

Instead of: yelling at your kids when they make an unwise or careless sexual decision.

Try saying: "I am going to love you no matter what, even when you make bad choices, and I'll always be here to help you deal with the consequences. I just hope that you can learn from this mistake and make better choices in the future."

Giving your kids guidelines for when sex is okay (as opposed to hard-and-fast rules) prepares them to make good sexual decisions for the rest of their lives, not just the first time they do it. They'll have the framework to decide if a relationship is worthy of sex, even after they're no longer virgins. Sex is something you want your kids to think about carefully every time. Each time matters, and each time counts. By helping them develop solid values around sexuality, you are giving them guidance that will last from their first love to their last. And the only thing that's as important as solid sexual values, is solid sexual safety habits.

Chapter Five SEXUALLY TRANSMITTED DISEASES

As kids go into adulthood, parents should take a proactive approach, and be knowledgeable about sexual health issues.

—Denniz Zolnoun, MD, OB-GYN, University of North Carolina at Chapel Hill

Shortly after I lost my virginity I went to my doctor for an annual checkup. For some reason or another he decided I might have gonorrhea (without even asking my sexual history), and told me he'd do a swab and get back to me in a week. Despite his complete nonchalance, and knowing nothing about gonorrhea myself, I completely flipped and called my mom hysterical from the parking lot convinced that my life was over. Luckily my mom, as a product of the 1960s, knew what was up. Even if I did have it (and as it turned out, I didn't), gonorrhea was completely curable and if caught early had no long-term repercussions. In retrospect, I feel lucky that I have a mother I can talk with about those sorts of things, but even more than that, I feel lucky to have a parent who's informed enough to help me through those sorts of situations.

There's no way around it, sexually transmitted diseases (STDs) are going to affect your child—whether it's because your daughter is getting the HPV (human papillomavirus) vaccine, your son gets cold sores and you have to explain the different types of herpes, or your teen actually contracts an STD. And because STDs will touch your children's life in some fashion, they are something you should know about and talk about with your kids.

To spare you the gory details of every STD imaginable, I've included an STD guide at the end of this book with specific details about the most common STDs (see Appendix A). This chapter is about the misconceptions many parents and teens have about STDs, some general sexual health points to discuss with your teen, and some pertinent details of the most common diseases.

Misconceptions about STDs

In order for teens to be able to make informed choices about sex, they must truly understand the risks involved. But because of widespread misconceptions about STDs, many teens underestimate those risks, and as a result, they have sex in situations they think are safe when they in fact are not. As a parent, the more you know about STDs, the better you can inform your teen about how to stay safe. The following are the most common misunderstandings many have about STDs.

I Won't Get an STD

The majority of teens have heard statistics about STDs. And most of those statistics are pretty shocking. According to many accounts, about half of all Americans will contract an STD by the time they are twenty-five (Cates et al. 2004). Each year there are at least 19 million new cases of STDs (Weinstock et al. 2004), and over half of all new HIV infections occur in young adults under twenty-five (UNAIDS 2008). But despite these high numbers, many teens just don't believe it could happen to them.

Most teens are shocked when they find out that they or someone they know has an STD. They think, "but she's so smart," "but he smells so good," "but she's so cute!" To many teens, STDs seem like something that happens to kids at other schools, who hang with a different crowd, or live in a different town. But "the kind of people who have STDs" are everywhere. And teens need to be reminded that STDs really can happen to everyone: rich, poor, hot, ugly, popular, geeky, their first boyfriend, their next girlfriend: really and truly *anyone*.

When Someone Has an STD, It's Obvious

You've probably seen pictures of STDs. They're probably the same pictures your child has seen: images of genitals so infected they look more like something you'd see snorkeling than something you'd see in between someone's legs: penises with collars of warts, vaginas with gaping sores, or unidentifiable genitals that kind of resemble conch shells. It's no mystery what feelings teachers are trying to evoke by showing these types of pictures: "STDs are gross, I don't want one." But those pictures are rare cases of people who probably don't have access to a doctor. And those horror stories are actually doing a disservice.

When teens see pictures like that, they assume that STDs are obvious—that they can pull down someone's pants and if his or her genitals aren't growing barnacles that person doesn't have an STD. But it's not that easy. The majority of people who have STDs don't show any signs or symptoms. And those who do often have symptoms that are very minor and could be mistaken for a small cut or ingrown hair. That's why STDs are spread so easily, because the people infected generally aren't aware of it.

REAL-LIFE ADVICE

Chances are, you regularly ask your child how his or her day went and inquire about different classes. To start talking about STDs, ask about your son or daughter's health class: "Has your health class shown you any crazy STD pictures? The really nasty ones where you can barely tell you're looking at a body part? Those pictures can be confusing because not all people with STDs have obvious signs. In fact, most don't. So you can't assume a person doesn't have an STD just because you don't see anything nasty when they take off their clothes. You also can't assume someone doesn't have an STD because they're really cute, the star of the football team, or the smartest girl in your grade. Really, *anyone* can have an STD. Anyone."

When you're talking with your teens about STDs, make sure they know that a visual inspection doesn't count as an STD test. That being said, of course, if they ever do encounter something funny, advise them to avoid the area.

If Someone Has "Been Tested" They're Fine

Many teens make the mistake of thinking they don't have to use a condom if they're having sex with someone who has "been tested." The tricky thing is, it's not always clear what "being tested" means. A guy or girl can easily be tested for chlamydia, gonorrhea, syphilis, and HIV. But for herpes and HPV, the "testing" isn't that simple.

There is a blood test for herpes, but it's not often used because people don't know what to do with the results. If someone has no sores or symptoms of herpes they don't want to get a blood test, discover they have the virus, and have to explain to all their future partners, I have herpes, but I've never had symptoms, so I don't know where in my body the virus is . . . and I don't know what that means for you. Much more often, someone will get tested for herpes only if he or she has a sore that the doctor can swab.

Testing for HPV (the virus that causes cervical cancer and genital warts) is especially problematic. There is no test a guy can get to determine if he's carrying the strain of HPV that causes cervical cancer in women. Women can get pap smears and HPV DNA tests to see if they have the cervical cancer strain of HPV—part of the reason that sexually active women are supposed to see their gynecologist on a regular basis. But as far as the strains of HPV that cause warts, there is no overall test for guys or girls (only a wart itself can be inspected). Someone who finds a bump that could be a genital wart has to get it visually diagnosed by a doctor. The doctor will look at the bump and decide if it's caused by HPV, if it's not caused by HPV, or if he just doesn't know. But since many people with the strain of HPV that can cause warts will never have a wart, they cannot be tested for this virus.

Long story short, the phrase "been tested" is more complicated than it sounds. Be sure your teen knows that if someone claims to have been "tested," the follow-up question needs to be "tested for what?" Not only is it uncommon for someone to have had every possible STD *test*, it's impossible for sexually active people to say for sure that they don't have an STD (since they may have HPV but just never had symptoms). That means your teen must understand that "tested" does not equal "no need for a condom."

Using a Condom Means Forgetting about STDs

Consistently using condoms is a very effective way to prevent spreading or contracting many STDs. It isn't, however, extremely effective at preventing *all* STDs. Here's why: STDs are spread one of two ways—through infected liquid coming into contact with a mucus membrane (eyes, nose, vagina, a guy's urethra, mouth, or anus) and through infected skin rubbing against skin. A condom's biggest strength is that if used correctly, it protects infected fluids (be it semen or vaginal discharge) from ever coming in contact with a membrane (most likely a mouth, vagina, urethra, or anus). That means that STDs like gonorrhea, chlamydia, HPV, and HIV can often be avoided through consistent condom use. A condom's biggest weakness is that it isn't biker shorts. STDs like genital warts, herpes, and syphilis can all cause sores around the groin, butt, upper thighs, and other places that aren't covered by a condom. For those STDs that are spread through skin coming into contact with skin, condoms just aren't fully protective.

Your kids should know it's always a good idea to use condoms, especially because they protect against the most devastating STD of all, HIV. But they should also know that even if they use a condom every time, they may still be at risk for contracting an STD. So no matter how diligent your teens may be about using protection, they still have to stay on top of their sexual health by visiting a doctor at the first sign of any sore, bump, or unusual genital symptom, and get tested when possible.

How People Get STDs

Generally, people get STDs through sexual contact, no surprise there. But it's important your kids understand that many different sex acts can put them at risk for STDs, not just penis-in-vagina intercourse.

One of the biggest misunderstandings teens have about how STDs are transmitted is that many consider oral sex to be safe sex. It's true, it's very unlikely for someone to get HIV from oral sex. Herpes, gonorrhea, syphilis, and HPV, on the other hand, can all be spread through oral sex. According to Linda Brown, MPH, Health Education Consultant at the South Carolina State Health Department, "Because HPV is so widespread, we're starting to see things we haven't really seen before. We're seeing teens with warts in their mouth, and young people with throat and neck cancer that is associated with HPV." Teens need to know that they can get STDs from oral sex and that when they have oral sex they should use a condom or an oral dam.

Another sex act teens may not think to use protection for is anal sex. Since anal sex won't lead to pregnancy, teens may not instinctively think to use a condom. But STD-wise, anal sex is actually more risky than vaginal sex because the membranes in the anus are thin, can be easily penetrated by STDs, and are more likely to tear during intercourse (allowing STDs direct access to the blood stream).

REAL-LIFE ADVICE

Next time you hear your teen mention the word "virgin," say this: "The whole idea of virginity is pretty tricky. You would think that a virgin can't have STDs. By many people's definition, someone who has only engaged in oral sex is a virgin. But you can get STDs from oral sex. You can get STDs from anal sex too. Hell, STDs like HPV you can even get by rolling around naked with someone. So even if someone is a 'virgin,' it doesn't mean that much in terms of their sexual health."

Perhaps the most confusing thing about STD transmission is that STDs can be spread through activities that teens might not consider to be sex acts at all. As mentioned earlier, some STDs are spread by skin-to-skin contact. So two people rolling around together naked are at risk for contracting an STD, even if technically no other sex act took place. The take-home message here is that to help teens understand their risks, they probably need to broaden their definition of "sex" and "sexually active." Very possibly, teens who consider themselves to be virgins may still be at risk for contracting an STD.

STD Basics

Sexually transmitted diseases aren't as straightforward as many people believe. Technically, pubic lice are considered an STD even though one can get them by sharing a towel with someone who's infected. Trichomoniasis can be passed through sexual contact, but most consider it to be a vaginal infection. Urinary tract infections are often brought on by sex, but again, not medically classified as an STD. So while the category of "sexually transmitted diseases" can actually include a variety of different infections, the main ones to keep on your radar are: genital herpes, HPV, gonorrhea, chlamydia, syphilis, and HIV.

The rest of this chapter includes a basic rundown of things you should know about these STDs. But first, these are the top six things you should know about STDs in general:

1. Many are curable. The term "sexually transmitted disease" makes it sound as though once you get one, you have it for the rest of your life (part of the reason many health care workers have started using the term STI—sexually transmitted infection). But many STDs are completely curable once they're caught. Gonorrhea, chlamydia, and syphilis can all be cured with antibiotics. So if detected, they aren't the worst thing in the world. But just because an STD is curable doesn't mean it's no big deal. All three of those STDs can wreak havoc on someone's body if undetected and left untreated. Gonorrhea and chlamydia are especially dangerous for young women because untreated infections can often lead to PID (pelvic inflammatory disease), which can permanently damage their reproductive systems, possibly causing chronic pelvic pain, infertility, and ectopic pregnancies. The CDC (Centers for Disease Control) estimates that 40 percent of the time a chlamydial infection is left untreated it will cause PID.
2. Someone may not get an STD on their first try. Just because a person is exposed to an STD doesn't mean he or she will necessarily get it. It may take several "tries" before a person actually contracts the virus or infection. For this

reason, it's important teens know that just because they had unprotected sex with a person once doesn't mean they may as well do it again. Each time a person has sex—even with the same partner—there is a new risk of contracting an STD if the partner is infected.

REAL-LIFE ADVICE

At some point when you're talking with your kids about decision making (even if it's not a conversation specifically about *sexual* decision-making), be sure to make the point that one bad decision doesn't have to lead to another. Tell them: "Even if you make a mistake and have unprotected sex, it doesn't mean that you've already messed up and you might as well keep having unprotected sex with that person. You won't necessarily contract an STD someone is carrying the first time. Each time there's a new risk, so even if you mess up once, it's still important to use a condom the next time."

3. Having or having recently had an STD makes someone more likely to get HIV. One complication with having some STDs, or even a vaginal infection, is that it makes someone more likely to get HIV if he or she is exposed and more likely to pass on HIV if he or she is infected.
4. The symptoms of STDs can be confusing. When someone has an STD, he or she won't necessarily be in that much discomfort. And for girls, STDs can be extra confusing because many have some of the same symptoms as common vaginal infections. I cannot tell you the number of

girls who have said the first time they had a yeast infection they thought it was an STD. But I can also imagine that there are many girls who have had an STD and didn't go to the doctor because they assumed it was a vaginal infection. For that reason, after the STD Guide at the end of this book is a Vaginal Infection Guide about all the nuances of common vaginal infections.

5. There are vaccines. There are vaccines for Hepatitis B and HPV. Hepatitis B is a very serious, life-threatening sexually transmitted disease that most children who regularly see a doctor get vaccinated against. The HPV vaccine is not quite as common, although it really should be. HPV is insanely widespread; according to some estimates, *at least* three-quarters of people will be exposed to it in their lifetime. The CDC now recommends the vaccine for girls, and considers it an option for boys as well. (For more information about the HPV vaccine, see the HPV section of this chapter.)
6. Girls are more likely to get an STD. STD-wise, not all's fair in love and warts. Because of the anatomy of things, a girl is significantly more likely to contract an STD from an act of unprotected sex than a guy. During intercourse, a vagina is more vulnerable than a penis. The vagina has a much larger surface area, and it's exposed to potentially disease-carrying fluids for a longer period of time (since after ejaculation the semen just sits there). Anyone—guy or girl—who is on the receiving end of anal sex is also more likely to get an STD than the guy who is the penetrator.

And now, for the diseases specifics you've all been waiting for . . .

HPV

The most important thing to know about HPV (human papillomavirus) is that you are in the unique position of being able to seriously reduce your child's chances of contracting it and passing it to someone else. But more about that later. First things first, HPV is the virus that causes cervical cancer and genital warts. There are over thirty strains of the virus that affect the genital area, and each strain has the potential to cause *either* warts or cervical cancer. However, warts do not turn into cervical cancer, and cervical cancer doesn't turn into warts. Any girl who has both symptoms is infected with two different strains of HPV at once. (Even if infected with multiple strains, a guy can only show symptoms for warts, since he doesn't have a cervix.)

TMI WARNING

It's important to explain to your teens that women (or the recipients of anal sex) are more vulnerable to STDs. Resist the urge, however, to demonstrate the anatomy with your hands—you know, the finger-in-the-fist gesture. Stick to the words "more vulnerable," and leave your hands in your pockets.

HPV is mind-blowingly common. As a gynecologist recently told me, "When you have sex with someone you're basically swapping strains of HPV, because you probably have it, and so does he." Because the genital warts strains of HPV are passed through skin-to-skin contact of the entire boxer shorts area, there's really no way to be sexually active and not potentially expose yourself to it. However, while the majority of sexually active people either have or have had HPV, many never show symptoms.

There's no cure for HPV, although doctors do believe that after a year or two the body will basically rid itself of the virus. In the meantime, the warts themselves or precancerous cells in the cervix *can* be treated.

Thanks to the miracles of medicine, there is now a vaccine for HPV, Gardasil (recommended for girls ages nine to twelve, or any woman who has not been vaccinated up to age twenty-six, and optional for boys). Gardasil protects against four strains of the virus. Four out of thirty may not seem impressive at first, but considering the fact that those four strains are responsible for 70 percent of cervical cancer cases, and 90 percent of genital warts cases, it's a vaccine parents should strongly consider for their children. The other thing you should consider is vaccinating boys as well. Even though a guy can't get cervical cancer, he can still carry HPV and give it to a girl he cares about. Giving your son the HPV vaccine not only ensures he won't pass on certain strains of the virus, it will also make him significantly less likely to ever develop genital warts. Maybe your kids aren't sexually active yet, but you know, at some point they will be. So if you have kids old enough to prompt you to be reading this book, you probably have kids old enough to get vaccinated.

What to tell your kids about HPV: "HPV is very common, and many people pass it on without even knowing they have it. You can be very sexually responsible and still get it, and the worst part about it is that it can cause cancer."

Herpes

According to the CDC, nearly one in four women and one in eight men in the United States have genital herpes. Herpes is a virus that can cause either blistery sores around the mouth or sores around the genitals. Many people are infected with herpes type 1 (the kind that most commonly causes cold sores) in childhood from simple kisses from infected family members. Herpes type 2 is sexually transmitted and generally causes genital sores. Sometimes, a partner with genital herpes can give their partner mouth sores from oral sex. Similarly, a partner with oral herpes can give their partner genital sores from oral sex.

Most often, genital herpes is passed through vaginal or anal intercourse. Using a condom greatly reduces one's risk of contracting herpes, but like HPV, since a condom doesn't cover the entire area that could have a sore, someone can still get herpes when using one. Another scary thing about herpes is that most people contract it from partners who don't know they have it, and have no visible sores. Although skin with an active sore is *more* contagious, skin with no visible symptoms can still carry the virus.

The worst thing about herpes is that a person who has it has it forever. It can't be cured, it doesn't leave the body, and outbreaks can continue for the rest of a person's life. The symptoms can, however, be managed with medication, and as time goes on, it's likely the outbreaks will become less frequent, and less painful.

What to tell your kids about herpes: "Even if you don't see any bumps, it doesn't necessarily mean a person doesn't have herpes or that they can't give it to you. And if you get herpes, you can treat your outbreaks, but you might have outbreaks for the rest of your life."

HIV/AIDS

Historically, HIV/AIDS was associated with gay men and drug users. But now, over a quarter of all new infections in the United States are in women—and young African American and Latina women are especially at risk. According to some estimates, half of all new HIV infections in the United States occur in young adults under twenty-five (although they may not discover it until years later).

HIV (human immunodeficiency virus) is the virus that attacks a person's T cells (necessary for a healthy immune system) and eventually causes AIDS (acquired immunodeficiency syndrome) if left unmanaged. People who are infected with HIV can seem completely healthy for years until they develop pneumonia or another AIDS-related disease and eventually die from the illness. Although there is no cure for HIV/AIDS, there are many drugs now available that can help HIV-infected people live longer and healthier lives.

A person can contract HIV by having unprotected vaginal or anal sex, but correctly using a condom significantly decreases a person's risk of contracting the virus. Although it's possible for a person to contract HIV through unprotected oral sex, it's really not that likely. Someone can't get HIV by hugging, kissing, sharing food with, sitting next to, or otherwise interacting with a person who is infected.

There are several different ways to get tested for HIV, and every sexually active person should get tested on a regular basis. Because the majority of the tests screen for the body's reaction to the HIV virus, people should wait at least two months after possible exposure before getting tested.

What to tell your kids about HIV: "New medications can do a lot to help people with HIV, but that doesn't mean that getting it is no big deal."

Chlamydia and Gonorrhea

Chlamydia is the most commonly reported bacterial STD in the United States. It's completely curable if caught early, but if left untreated in a girl, it can permanently damage her reproductive system causing infertility, pregnancy complications, and chronic pelvic pain. While antibiotics will cure chlamydia no matter how long the infection has been in a person's body, any damage it has done cannot be reversed. The best way to detect a chlamydia infection is to test for it. Since only about half of men and a quarter of women actually have symptoms (burning when peeing, itching in the genital area, or an abnormal discharge), a person who has had unprotected sex should get tested even if he or she feels fine.

SAY NO TO DOUCHE BAGS

Tell your daughter not to douche. Not only can douching mask the symptoms of gonorrhea or chlamydia, it can also spread the infection to other organs.

Gonorrhea is very much like chlamydia in that it's a bacterial sexually transmitted disease with similar symptoms, and it's treatable with antibiotics. It's not quite as common as chlamydia, but can permanently damage both men's and women's reproductive systems if left untreated. Sexually active people can get gonorrhea in virtually any orifice of their bodies: their genitals, their mouth, their anus, or their throat, and the best way to discover an infection is to test for it. Interestingly, people who test positive for gonorrhea, often have chlamydia as well, so many doctors will treat someone for both gonorrhea and chlamydia if a gonorrheal infection is discovered.

What to tell your kids about gonorrhea and chlamydia: "Gonorrhea and chlamydia are the easiest STDs to test for. And if either of these is caught early you can treat it and be fine. But if a girl doesn't discover an infection and treat it properly it can destroy her reproductive organs."

Hepatitis B

As mentioned earlier, Hepatitis B is a potentially life-threatening STD that your child can avoid completely if he or she gets vaccinated (and chances are your child already has been). Since the full three-shot vaccination should ideally be completed before someone becomes sexually active, adolescents should get it sooner rather than later. If there is any doubt in your mind about whether or not your children have been vaccinated, have their doctor check their immunizations records.

Syphilis

Syphilis is a fairly uncommon bacterial STD, but recently rates have been rising in certain populations. Gay and bisexual men, African Americans, and people in the southeastern United States are at the highest risk for contracting this STD. If detected, it is completely treatable, but if left untreated it can cause a variety of health complications and even be fatal.

STD Info to Give Your Teen Cheat Sheet

Here's a summary of STD information covered in this chapter that you should talk about with your teen.

1. Anyone can get an STD, and many sexually active people will (50–75 percent of Americans, depending on the estimate).
2. The signs and symptoms of STDs often aren't obvious, which is why you can't know for sure if someone has an STD unless they've been tested. But the tricky thing is that tests for every type of STD aren't always available.

3. Genital warts and herpes can be spread just by rolling around naked with someone. And since they can affect the entire "boxer shorts area," even someone who uses a condom isn't fully protected.
4. Gonorrhea, chlamydia, and syphilis can all be treated with antibiotics, but if left untreated can cause permanent damage to a person's body.
5. Just because a person is exposed to an STD doesn't necessarily mean he or she will get it the first time around. Anyone who has an STD or vaginal infection may be more likely to get HIV if exposed.
6. Because of anatomy, women (or those on the receiving end of anal sex) are more likely to contract an STD. Also of concern to girls, many STDs mirror symptoms of common vaginal infections.
7. There is now a vaccine for certain strains of HPV. The HPV vaccine protects people against four strains of HPV. Together, those four strains are responsible for 70 percent of cervical cancer cases and 90 percent of genital warts cases.

Chapter Six CONDOMS AND SAFER SEX

I swear the first time I heard my mom say the word "penis" was last week. My dad was in the hospital and had a stent in. My mom explained to me, "they will have to remove it through his penis." I almost died when she said that!

—Kerry, age forty-four

Condoms: they're an absolute necessity. But using one every time with every partner is a goal that's beyond challenging for many teens (and many adults). The problem with condoms and other forms of barrier protection (orals dams and female condoms) is that they have to be used during the heat of the action. That means having the will power to not get swept up in the moment—and most teens aren't a fan of that practical reality.

TMI WARNING

In order to address all of your teens' possible condom concerns you are going to have to flirt with crossing the line of being a bit too graphic. But after weighing the mortification factor (for both you and them) against your children's sexual health, guess what, their health won. So while I realize that the suggested dialogs and the activities in this section may make you a bit uncomfortable, I do believe they are necessary. If you have the option though, it might be a good idea to have the same-sex parent or a same-sex older relative initiate these conversations.

As a parent, one of the best things you can do for your children's sexual health is to convince them it's stupid to make "the moment" a bigger priority than the rest of their life. Help them understand that no matter what hesitation they or their partner may have about using protection, it's a much smaller deal than the potential of contracting an STD or becoming pregnant. The goal of this chapter is to help you teach your kids to have positive attitudes about condoms (and other forms of barrier contraception), and to be able to deal with any opposition they may face to using one. But this chapter is also about safer sex in a broader sense—because safe sex is more than just knowing how to use a condom. It's about helping your teens stand up for themselves and their sexual health, and teaching them how to get out of unsafe and uncomfortable sexual situations.

Condoms

In terms of access, there's really no reason sexually active teens shouldn't always be prepared with a stash of condoms. They can buy them at drugstores, gas stations, Planned Parenthood offices, grocery stores, and even pick them up for free at some health centers. It's good for teens to keep condoms around, since studies show (unsurprisingly) that when there's a condom immediately available, teens are significantly more likely to use one. Studies also show that just because condoms are available, it doesn't make kids any more likely to have sex (Blake et al. 2003). Trust me, in all the people I've talked to about sexual choices, I have *never* heard of someone deciding to have sex just because they had a condom.

You want to do everything in your power to make sure your kids use condoms. But more than that, you want your kids to use them correctly (otherwise they aren't as effective). It may have been some time since you've had to deal with condoms, so you might feel a bit unprepared to show them how to use one. For this reason, the next few pages are a breakdown of the correct way to use a condom. Some of these steps may seem obvious to you. But things that are intuitive to you could be groundbreaking intelligence for your teen. So like everything else that has to do with sex, it's important to give your children detailed information—even if at times what you're saying seems obvious.

Store Them Correctly and Check the Date

Ideally, condoms should be stored at around room temperature. This means glove compartments, wallets, and purses aren't the best storage spots—at least on a long-term basis. Although it's fine to put a condom in a backpack or bag for a date that evening, the main stash should be somewhere inside, in a climate-controlled environment, and where it's not getting sat on, tumbled around, or otherwise mangled.

What comes as a surprise to many teens is that condoms have an expiration date clearly marked on the package—meaning a person has to make sure the condom is "still good." It also means that if you bought your son a giant box of "just in case" condoms when he hit puberty, don't send them with him to college, because they've likely expired. Condoms that are past date or stored in extreme temperatures are much more likely to break. But an improperly stored/out of date condom is *always* better than no condom at all.

Put It On Before the Action Starts

For condoms to most effectively prevent STDs they need to be put on before there is any contact between the penis and the vagina (or the penis and any other orifice). "Using a condom" doesn't mean two people rubbing their genitals together then putting on a condom before there is full penetration. "Using a condom" means preventing the penis and vagina from ever touching. Since many STDs are passed through skin-to-skin contact, starting to use one halfway though sex doesn't provide enough protection. Teens need to understand that once underwear comes off, a condom should go on.

Treat Condoms with Care and Lubricate Them Correctly

Teach your kids to be delicate when opening condoms. Biting open or ferociously ripping the package can rip the condom along with the wrapper (hey, who knows what one might do in the heat of the moment). Also tell your teen that only water-based lubricants, like K-Y Jelly, can be used with a condom. Oil-based lubricants like Vaseline, many lotions, massage oil, or anything that can be found in a kitchen can weaken the latex.

Pinch and Roll

The point of the bump at the tip of the condom is to collect the semen that comes out of the penis, not to be a cute balloon. If the tip is filled with air, the condom is more likely to pop open. To prevent that from happening, it's imperative to pinch the tip before rolling the condom down the shaft of the penis. You may also want to clarify that a condom must be put on an erect penis, not a flaccid one.

When You're Done, Get Outta There!

As soon as the guy has finished, he must hold the base of the condom and withdraw. Continuing to have sex after ejaculation will loosen the condom (as he's losing his erection), and push the semen down toward the edge (where it could slip out into the vagina). To keep the condom from slipping off as he's withdrawing, a guy should grip the base of it to ensure that it comes out with his penis. A condom slipping off after sex isn't as unusual a problem as you might think. So while telling your kids to grip the base while pulling out may seem a bit excessive, it's a necessary precaution.

Throw It Away

Condoms are meant to be used once and only once. Once a condom has been unrolled, it's as good as used, whether or not it has been ejaculated in. Guys cannot have sex (not ejaculate), keep the condom on for the next hour or so, then get another erection and go at it again. Only one condom per boner, please.

In a way, using a condom is kind of like flying an airplane. If something is going to go wrong, it's probably going to happen during takeoff or landing, not because of turbulence during the flight. As long as one is cognizant while putting a condom on and taking one off, both parties can relax and enjoy the ride.

Fun for the Whole Family!

Okay, not the *whole* family. But it's probably a good idea to corner your teen with a banana and a handful of condoms and teach him or her the right way to use them. To cut down on the mortification factor, do your condom lesson with just you and your teen; don't bring up the idea or give the lesson in front of their friends (unless they want you to), siblings, or extended family. Explain the important parts of condom use: keeping them handy (but in a climate controlled stationary environment when possible), checking the date, putting one on *before* the action starts, opening them gently, using a water-based lubricant, pinching the tip, stopping after ejaculation, grabbing the base when withdrawing, and throwing the condom away. It's a lot of steps to remember, so you may want to simplify it by remembering: before any action starts, get a condom then check it, pinch it, grab it, trash it.

Asking to Use a Condom

Believe it or not, some teens find talking about sex with a partner awkward—hard to imagine what sort of society would instill that value! And for teens who find talking about sex awkward, asking to use a condom isn't the easiest thing in the world. Many teens find it easier to just start having sex than to verbally confirm it's about to happen by talking about condoms. Knowing this, talk with your teen about how to discuss using a condom with a partner. That way, he or she will have had time to think about it beforehand and be better prepared.

In order to be helpful, you have to offer realistic suggestions. As much as you may want to tell your children to demand that a condom be used, suggesting they say, "Get a condom" just isn't realistic. Talking about condoms is tricky because "Should I get a condom?" has become somewhat synonymous with "Do you want to have sex?" And because of that, wordings like "I'm getting a condom," or "Go get a condom," sound both presumptuous and aggressive. If it were standard practice for teens to ask, "Do you want to have sex?" then following up with a demand about a condom would be fine. But since that doesn't usually happen, the majority of teens feel most comfortable using phrases along the lines of "Should I get a condom," or "Do you want to get a condom?" Essentially, any phrase that asks a question as opposed to makes a demand.

What If They Say "No"?

It's very possible that one day your teen will be with a partner who doesn't want to use a condom—whether it's a guy who doesn't like the way condoms feel, a girl who thinks using a condom is less intimate, or a partner who feels insulted that using a condom insinuates he or she has an STD. There are a few ways a teen might want to respond to that reaction. One is to remind the partner that protection is a two-way street, and say, "Using a condom protects you too." Another is to appeal to the partner's ego and say, "I won't enjoy sex unless we use one." (Even selfish people usually want to look good in the bedroom.) Remind your kids that, ultimately, actions speak louder than words. Any person who refuses to use a condom after being asked to either doesn't care about the relationship or is too selfish to be in one.

Something all teens should be reminded of is that they can always just get up and walk away. We spend so much time drilling it into kids' heads they should "finish what they've started," that many view sex the same way. It's very possible that the idea of leaving a sexual situation if they feel uncomfortable (because of a condom disagreement or otherwise) may have never occurred to them.

It's especially important for girls to know it's okay to leave a sexual situation. Girls grow up hearing about "blue balls" and thinking that the worst thing you can do to a guy is let him get turned on and then not get him off. But in reality, "blue balls" don't occur nearly as often as you might think. Yes, if a guy is literally about to have an orgasm and then doesn't it is possible for him to feel an aching sensation in his testicles. However, guys do not get blue balls just from having a boner and then not getting off. And even if a guy does get them, the sensation will go away as soon as he ejaculates. Honestly, I've watched teen guys punch each other in the crotch for a laugh—clearly they can't be that adverse to a little testicular pain.

When to Tell Your Teen to Lie

No one wants to raise a liar. But in the real world, teens can end up in sexual situations where they may have trouble asserting themselves or voicing their true concerns. And while you hope your kids will always have the strength to stand up for themselves, it's possible that sometimes they won't. In those situations, it's important they have a safety net. Because at the end of the day, someone's sexual health trumps the importance of always telling the truth. The following are a few white lies I'd encourage your kids to tell.

1. **"I had this condom for a friend"/"Someone gave it to me as a joke."** Some teens worry that carrying a condom makes it look like they're expecting sex. That concern then gets in the way of a teen always being prepared. You should explain that having a condom just makes someone

look responsible and sends the message a person is on top of their sexual health. But if your kids aren't quite sold on being prepared, give them the previous excuse to help seal the deal.

2. **"I'm on/about to start my period."** Clearly, this isn't an excuse that's going to work for a guy. But any girl who is unwilling to speak up about being uncomfortable in a sexual situation that is making her uncomfortable can always use the excuse of her period. Or she can say that she's about to start it and is afraid that if she had sex the guy's penis might come out bloody. As I remember from high school, nothing can stop a guy in his tracks like the threat of a little blood.
3. **"I have to be home"/"My parents could come home any minute."** This excuse can be a good one for guys to use if they want out of a sexual situation. Because culturally we expect guys to "take it when they can get it," it's often much more difficult for a guy (especially as a teen) to say he doesn't want to have sex. But any teen—guy or girl—who is in the middle of a sexual encounter in their own house can always use the excuse: "My parents could get home any minute." Teens who are out somewhere can say: "I need to get home now or I'm going to be grounded." Another possibility is to set up a code word with your kids, and if they ever call you and say the word it will be your cue to tell them they need to come home immediately.

In any uncomfortable or unsafe sexual situation the first priority is for teens to be able to get out. Afterward, they can think about how to better assert themselves in the future and why they couldn't be straightforward with their partner at the time. They might also want to consider what they can do to keep themselves out of uncomfortable situations all together. Maybe that means getting to know partners better before spending time alone with them, or only entering sexual relationships with people who have already proven to be concerned with their comfort and needs. But no matter what strategy they come up with, be sure your kids know that they can always use you as an excuse.

Complaints about Condoms

Although the threat of STDs may have some teens alarmed, many just don't believe it could happen to them, or they refuse to think their clean, good-looking significant other could have one. And because so many teens underestimate their risk of contracting an STD, instead of feeling thankful for condoms, they complain about them. There are hundreds of excuses teens may cite as reasons why they didn't—or don't like to—use condoms. But usually, they all boil down to the same general complaints. The better you can anticipate and address the problems your teen may have with condom use, the more likely your teen will be to use one. In order to help your teen consistently use condoms, you have to counter these concerns:

Sex with Condoms Doesn't Feel as Good

Coming from guys, this one is a no-brainer: condoms can reduce the sensation that men feel during sex. But surprisingly, I find that girls complain about the way condoms feel equally as much. Some girls don't like the sensation of rubbing against latex, and others feel their vaginas get irritated from the lubrication on the condoms.

You can counter this complaint by suggesting to your son that he buy ultrathin condoms, or that he try out a few different brands, since they may all feel different. Depending on the relationship you have with him, and if you're feeling bold, you can always remind him that girls enjoy sex that lasts longer—so that perhaps it's *good* that condoms reduce what he feels. There's nothing like a blow to a guy's sexual prowess to help him see condoms in a more positive light.

A suggestion you can make to your daughter is that she buy nonlubricated condoms, and use K-Y Jelly if she needs extra lubrication. Lubricated condoms, particularly condoms lubricated with spermicide, can be irritating for many girls. A few girls (and guys) may actually be allergic to latex, and in that case, they can buy special polyurethane condoms, which aren't as effective as latex condoms but are still better than no condom at all.

TMI WARNING

You need to address the reduced pleasure issue when talking about condoms, but there's no need to get overly detailed or beat a dead horse here. The conversation shouldn't go like this: "You might worry about a guy's sexual pleasure being reduced by using a condom, that he won't have the same friction as rubbing up against a vagina bareback, and that he'll have a harder time coming. . . ."

Sex with Condoms Doesn't Feel as Good for My Partner

About half of all teens—both guys and girls—agree that one of the main reasons contraception isn't used during sex is because their partner doesn't want to use it (The National Campaign to Prevent Teen and Unplanned Pregnancy 2000). I think this concern is especially relevant to young women. Girls who feel insecure in a relationship, or think that a guy's sexual pleasure is more important than their own, might not demand a condom be used because they want their partner to "fully enjoy" sex.

Counter this complaint by reminding your teen that millions of people use condoms everyday and still have enjoyable experiences. Also remind them that sexual health always trumps sexual pleasure, and tell your daughter that no guy will like her more just because she didn't make him use a condom. Most important, explain to your teens that any partner who cares about them will care about their enjoyment too. If someone is only concerned with his or her own sexual pleasure, that's not the kind of person you should be dating or sleeping with anyway.

REAL-LIFE ADVICE

As you're talking to your teen about the importance of condoms or how to use one, make sure you throw in this advice: "You should never be worried that asking someone to use a condom will affect the way that person feels about you. If a partner cares about you, he/she will be happy to use a condom if you want to. Your partner should care about making you comfortable, and if not, that's not someone you should be with."

Having Sex with a Condom Makes It Less Intimate

This issue comes up the most within couples: young adults in long-term monogamous relationships don't like the idea of using a condom *every* time they have sex. Understandably, no one thinks his or her Boo has STDs, so using a condom within a relationship can seem less critical.

Counter this complaint by telling your teens that using a condom when having sex with someone they care about can be an expression of just how much they care. Every time a condom is used, both people are protected. Tell them that since they would never want to harm their partner in any way, they should insist on using a condom—not just for their own protection, but for their partner's. In that vein, using a condom can make sex *more* intimate.

Using a Condom Is Insulting and Emasculating

Most teens view condom use primarily as a way to prevent STDs rather than a way to prevent pregnancy. While STD prevention is exactly why many teens use condoms, ironically it's also why many do not. It's not uncommon for teens to refuse to ask their partner to use a condom because they feel that request implies their partner has an STD. According to Andrew Drucker, an Algebra teacher in the Bronx public school system, a lot of his male students feel condoms are emasculating. They think, "Condoms are for gay couples to prevent AIDS . . . that's not how I roll." For groups of teens who feel condom use carries a negative connotation, getting them to use a condom is especially hard. If they don't believe using a condom is a good idea to begin with, it's highly unlikely they'll decide to use one in the heat of the moment.

Counteract this concern by creating a positive attitude about condoms in your house. Tell your teen that everyone: rock stars, athletes, rap artists, and other celebrities use condoms all the time. Condoms are a very effective way to protect people from both pregnancy and STDs. Explain to your teen, "Asking to use a condom shouldn't be insulting; it shows your partner you're confident enough to state your feelings, smart enough to know your risks, and looking out for your sexual health."

REAL-LIFE ADVICE

After you've had some initial conversations about condoms or STDs, start to talk with your teen about some of his or her condom concerns. Say, "You know, whenever we've talked about condoms, we've never talked about the things people don't like about them. Some people think that asking someone to use a condom might be insulting or that using one is less intimate. But the way I see it, using a condom just shows how much you care, how responsible you are, and how seriously you take the relationship. It's not saying, 'I think you have an STD,' it's saying, 'I want to protect us both from STDs and an unplanned pregnancy.' And if you're ever that worried about offending your partner by asking to use a condom, you can always tell a white lie and say, 'The only reason I want to use one is for pregnancy protection.'"

Putting on a Condom Is Disruptive

Very often teens who planned on using a condom don't because they don't want to disrupt the action by stopping to put one on. Many teens aren't comfortable handling condoms, and feel like the whole process of putting one on is a fumbling mess and a mood killer.

Counter this complaint by telling your teen: "Putting on a condom takes about five seconds. Taking off a bra, getting out of boxers (especially if a guy is lying down), or taking off a sweater can all take much longer than that. But you wouldn't have sex fully clothed because it takes too much time to get naked."

The truth is, putting on a condom isn't any more disruptive than many other things that have to be done before having sex. The only difference is that while teens look at getting undressed as part of sex, they see condom use as a disruption from it. Tell your kids to think of using a condom as just another part of sex (like getting naked), and that way it will feel less disruptive to use one.

Condoms Are Awkward

Many people find the act of putting on a condom awkward. Some feel weird sitting there doing nothing while their partner is putting one on. And others feel uneasy putting one on their partner or putting one on in front of their partner. Guys wonder: "Am I just supposed to stand here proudly with my boner?" And girls wonder: "Am I supposed to stare lustfully as he unrolls the protective sheath onto his magic wand?"

Counter this complaint by explaining first of all that sex *is* awkward—especially at the beginning. So they feel awkward using a condom. Well, you know what, I'd guess they feel awkward at other points too. Sex is messy, embarrassing, and not always all that sexy. Since condom use is part of sex, by default it can feel awkward too, but that's not the condom's fault.

You can then offer teens the advice that they might feel less awkward when putting on a condom if they continue to touch and kiss their partner, instead of just stopping the action come condom time.

The more practice teens have handling condoms the more comfortable they will feel using one (hence the condom activity I suggested earlier). They won't feel uneasy about the physical process of putting one on because they'll know which way the condom unrolls, what it feels like, and how to put it on.

At the end of the day, feeling really self-conscious about any aspect of sex should make your teen stop and think. If condom use is that awkward, it's probably a sign someone isn't comfortable enough with their partner to be sleeping with him or her in the first place. My golden rule of awkward condom use to girls is this: if you feel awkward looking at a guy's penis while he puts on a condom, or touching a guy's penis with your hand while you put a condom on him, then you are going to feel *real* awkward when his penis is in your vagina! (And that same advice—only vice versa—can be given to guys.)

REAL-LIFE ADVICE

Next time you're with your teen and there is a sex scene on TV or in a movie, explain to him or her what real sex is like. Say, "When people have sex it doesn't look as good as it does in the movies, and isn't as magical as people often make it out to be. Sex can be messy, there can be funny noises, and parts can feel pretty unsexy and awkward. You know, it's funny, some people complain that it feels awkward to use a condom, but it's really not any more awkward—heck probably less—than many other things that happen during sex."

Condoms aren't perfect. Yes, they reduce sensation; yes, they take a second to put on; and yes, there are probably a million other downsides your teen will think up. But your ace in the hole on this one is that unprotected sex is *never* the right choice. Years down the road, your teen isn't going to be reflecting on his or her life thinking: "You know what, I'm happy where I'm at now; things are good. But if I had just had a little more unprotected sex. Just a little. I think I'd be better off." With all the unknowns we face in life, walking into a situation knowing—with 100 percent certainty—that using a condom is the right way to go, that's a pretty solid argument for protected sex. You may regret a relationship, you may regret a sex act, but no one ever regrets using a condom.

Female Condoms

Male condoms aren't the only choice your teen has for STD protection during intercourse; there are female condoms. But on the whole, female condoms aren't the best choice for barrier protection. They are harder to find, harder to use, and not as effective. Realistically, they just aren't used that much—as many college students as I've spoken with about sex, I've never spoken to anyone who uses female condoms. But to be fair, if female condoms were given as much national attention as male condoms (in pop culture, education programs, and health initiatives), I imagine they would be used more often.

Female condoms *can* be the best choice for STD protection for some people. Anyone who is in a relationship with a guy who will not wear a condom (or refuses to ask a guy to wear a condom) can still protect herself (and him) by using a female condom. Female condoms can also be used in the anus, so gay men who are encountering issues with male condom use have the option of using a female condom during anal sex. Female condoms can also be good for people with latex allergies because unlike most male condoms, they are made of polyurethane.

If you bring up the topic of female condoms with your kids, make sure they know it's not extra protective to use a male condom *and* a female condom at the same time. Although that may initially seem like a bright idea, if used at the same time, they get tangled up in one another and become completely ineffective.

Very likely, you've never even seen a female condom, let alone know how to use one. Basically, it's a plastic pouch with a ring on either end (almost like a larger version of an unrolled male condom). To use it, a girl pinches the closed end of the condom and sticks it all the way up her vagina. The open end then hangs out about an inch below her vaginal opening. (If a guy is using the condom for anal sex, he inserts it the same way, but into his anus). When sex first starts a guy must be careful that his penis is actually going into the pouch, not between the pouch and the vagina. After sex is finished, the condom can be pulled out by grabbing the outer ring. And just like a male condom, it must be thrown away.

Oral Dams

For oral sex on a girl, teens have the option of using an oral dam (dental dam) to prevent the spread of STDs. But in all honesty, oral dam use just isn't that common. Under the "interests" section of my Facebook page I included "oral dams" in a long list of sexual health topics. A lesbian friend of mine saw that and wrote on my wall, "Thanks for the oral dam shout out, but does anyone actually use those?" Though common or not, they are an effective way to prevent transmitting STDs during oral sex on a girl.

Perhaps one of the reasons that oral dam use is so rare is that they're nearly impossible to find. You can't buy them in gas stations and grocery stores, and only some drug stores carry them. Planned Parenthood offices or online retailers are probably the best places to get one. But all issues of finding one aside, using one is incredibly simple.

An oral dam is simply a sheet of latex, and to use it, a person places it over the vaginal area so that the mouth and the vagina never make direct contact. Oral dams do come dusted in powder, and some people like to rinse it off before using it, but a person doesn't have to. The most important thing to tell your teen about using an oral dam is to keep one side on the vagina, the other side on the mouth, and not switch it up. If the dam gets flipped over, then fluids from the vagina are coming into contact with the mouth and vice versa. Make sure your teen also knows that oral dams can only be used once, they're not a rinse and reuse type of tool (even though they kind of look like they could be). And a quick tip, if a teen wants to use protection but can't find an oral dam, plastic wrap works just as well.

BARRIER PROTECTION CHEAT SHEET

Here's a summary of the topics covered in this chapter, and the major issues/questions to discuss with your kids:

1. If there's any chance you could be having sex, keep a condom on you.
2. How to use a condom: Check it, pinch it, grab it, trash it.
3. Have you thought about how you would ask your partner to use a condom?
4. A partner who cares about you will respect your needs, want you to enjoy sex, and therefore be happy to use a condom if you ask.
5. All sorts of people use condoms everyday and still enjoy sex.
6. There are ways to make putting on a condom less disruptive, and make protected sex more physically pleasurable.
7. Putting on a condom takes no more time than taking off your clothes, and if you feel really uncomfortable about using one, it could be a sign you're not ready to have sex (or not ready to have sex with that partner).
8. Do you worry about offending someone by asking him or her to use a condom?

9. If you're uncomfortable in a sexual situation, it's always okay to get up and leave or make up a white lie.
10. You will never regret your decision to use a condom!
11. You also have the option of using a female condom during sex or anal sex, or an oral dam during oral sex on a girl.

Chapter Seven CONTRACEPTION

Talking to your teens about birth control is not the same as giving them permission to have sex—and they won't see it that way. It tells teens that you think they're mature enough to make an important decision to protect their future, and that you want them to have good information

—Katharine O'Connell White, MD, MPH, OB-GYN at Tufts University–Baystate Medical Center

Ideally, young women would be psyched about the fact that by taking a pill, they can have sex and avoid pregnancy—OMG, the miracles of modern-day medicine! But in reality, many girls see the pill as something that will make them fat, bitchy, and perpetually nauseous. And although there are lots of other birth control options, most girls either aren't aware of them or automatically assume the worst.

Girls need to stop hating contraception. Condoms are a great way to protect against the spread of STDs, but when it comes to pregnancy prevention, they just don't cut it. Sexually active young women need to be on a contraceptive method even if they're planning on using condoms. And as their gatekeeper to the health care system, part of your responsibility is to make sure they are.

In order for you to help your daughter find a method of contraception that's best suited for her, you need be informed yourself. You have to know what rumors are swirling around about different methods, what her options are, and how to be the most useful in a health care setting. This chapter includes everything you need to know about contraception in order to best help your daughter make informed choices.

The Beef with Birth Control

The way young women badmouth contraception, you would think it had slept with all of their boyfriends. Girls love to hate birth control: blaming it for weight gain, causing cancer, infertility, relationship problems, and more. No birth control method is without side effects, that much is true. But as far as the severity of the side effects, many are blown completely out of proportion.

All of girls' contraceptive concerns wouldn't be such a roadblock if girls were actually afraid of getting pregnant. After all, what's a little hormonal oversensitivity compared to an unplanned pregnancy? But the problem is that many girls just don't believe it will happen to them. Every girl I know who's gotten pregnant has told me that even though she was aware of the statistics, she was still shocked when it actually happened to her. For many girls, the thought of becoming pregnant just doesn't penetrate into their reality. According to a 2007 survey, 45 percent of teen girls admit they've never really thought about what life would be like if they got pregnant as a teen (The National Campaign to Prevent Teen and Unplanned Pregnancy).

In order to effectively motivate your daughter to use contraception, you have to address her concerns (even if those concerns seem unimportant or silly to you). You can't soothe her worries with one fell swoop of, "Well it's better than being pregnant," because for many girls pregnancy doesn't seem like a realistic threat.

The following are some of the misconceptions girls have about contraception:

Myth #1
Hormonal Contraception Will Make Me Fat

FACT: As many women lose weight on the pill as gain.

A high school friend once told me that if she could have one wish in the entire world it would be to lose five pounds. Not a new car, not a hot boyfriend, not a million dollars . . . five pounds. Sure, she was more concerned about her body than many girls, but every girl I know thinks about her weight, and most have thought about it since high school. So for the girls who believe that birth control makes you gain, going on hormonal contraception isn't an option they want to consider.

But despite the common fear of gaining weight as a result of going on the pill, research suggests that isn't any more likely to happen than *losing* weight after going on the pill. The problem is, for many teens, friends' stories speak louder than the facts. If your daughter's friend Kimmy started taking birth control pills and gained ten pounds, "what the research says" isn't going to be a strong enough case to counteract what she witnessed firsthand.

If your daughter is wary of hormonal contraception because of her friend's experience, help her think rationally about what else could have caused the weight gain. Often girls will start taking birth control pills when they have a serious boyfriend. And maybe having that boyfriend means having meals with him at all of his favorite fast-food joints around town. Very often, a girl beginning birth control pills coincides with another event in her life: going away to college, having a boyfriend, or getting older (when a girl's body starts to fill out on its own). Just because a girl on birth control gained weight doesn't necessarily mean it's the birth control that caused it.

Myth #2
Birth Control Will Turn Me into a Hormonal Mess

FACT: The right contraception shouldn't affect a girl's mood *that* much.

Many girls say they're afraid that if they start using hormonal contraception they'll go completely wacko. I know a girl who refuses to take birth control pills because she thinks it will make her irrational (even though she's never tried taking them). Her boyfriend had a previous girlfriend who blamed her moodiness on the pill, and ever since then, he doesn't want the girls he dates to be putting hormones in their bodies. My friend tells me, "It's so relieving that when we fight and I start crying, I know it's not because of my pill but because I'm actually upset."

The truth is, the majority of girls should be able to find a birth control pill that doesn't make them feel emotionally unstable. There are currently sixty-nine different brands on the market, with different hormone combinations and doses. If a girl feels off kilter on one pill, she can always switch to another, or to another type of contraception all together, until she finds one she likes. However, it will always be easier for a girl to blame a pill for her relationship problems rather than confronting the real source—her boyfriend.

Myth #3
Hormonal Contraception Causes Cancer

FACT: The latest research suggests hormonal contraception does not cause cancer.

Studies show birth control pills actually make women less likely to get endometrial and ovarian cancer. Breast cancer is the only type of cancer thought to occur more often in women who take hormonal contraception, but even that claim is now being challenged. According to the most recent research, women who take hormonal contraception are not anymore likely to get breast cancer than those who don't. But if your daughter is concerned about this risk, she can talk about it with her physician before she goes on birth control.

Myth #4
IUDs Make Women Infertile

FACT: The new IUD is completely safe.

The reputation of the Dalkon Shield of the 1970s, which caused infertility in a number of women, has forever blackened the reputation of the intrauterine device (IUD). Baystate Medical Center OB-GYN Katharine O'Connell White is shocked when fourteen-year-olds show up in her office and say they don't want to use an IUD, "the T," because they don't want to become infertile. "They weren't even born when the Dalkon Shield was out. How could they possibly hear this?" The IUDs available to young women these days are completely safe, very effective, easy to use, and the most widely used birth control method around the world (in countries where there isn't a stigma). Many health care providers I speak with believe this is actually the best method of birth control for many teens.

When dealing with any concern your daughter may have about contraception, it's important to remember two things: one, just because it happened to her friend doesn't mean it will happen to her, and two, if she doesn't like one form of contraception she can always switch to another or stop all together.

REAL-LIFE ADVICE

If you hear your daughter talking about what one type of hormonal contraception did to one of her friends make sure you chime in: "You know that everyone's body is different. And just because one of your friends didn't like a certain kind of birth control, that doesn't mean that you wouldn't like it too. And even if one of your friends gets pregnant while using one type of birth control, it doesn't mean that kind is bad—no method is perfect."

Although personal stories will always seem more relevant than "what the research says," your daughter has to keep in mind that her body is different from her friend's. Just because someone she knew had a bad reaction to a type of contraception, it doesn't mean she will too. Just as people come in different shapes and sizes on the outside, they're different on the inside as well.

The fear of a possible bad reaction shouldn't stop a girl from trying a certain kind of contraception. Many side effects that may be present initially go away after a few months, and if there is anything that intolerable, she can always stop the method all together. Make sure your daughter also knows about all of the *positive* side effects of contraception that don't go away: clearer skin, more regular periods, less cramping, and lighter flow just to name a few. Not to mention of course, the bonus of having sex without having to worry as much about becoming pregnant. Even if your daughter isn't planning on having sex in the near future, make sure she knows that when she does, there are many contraceptive options available, with very moderate side effects.

Different Contraceptive Options

These days, there are many different forms of contraception available to young women, and no one option is the best for everyone. No option is perfect either, but with regular doctor visits nearly all young women should be able to find one that's tolerable. In the advice of Gretchen S. Stuart, a gynecologist at the University of North Carolina at Chapel Hill, "Girls should have an understanding of all of their options and know that they are all safe to use. From there, it's just a matter of determining which method will fit their life style and side effect tolerance the best." The following are some brief descriptions of different methods of contraception. Along with the descriptions, I've highlighted the pros and cons that separate some of the choices from each other. While I don't expect you to memorize all this information, I do think it's helpful to have a basic understanding of the options available. Ultimately, however, remember, it is your *daughter* who will have to choose the method that will work best for her.

"The Pill"

PROS: Birth control pills can help regulate a girl's period, decrease menstrual cramps, and clear up her skin.

CONS: You have to remember to take it every day, and some girls may experience nausea, irregular bleeding, mood changes, or other side effects.

"The pill" (i.e., oral contraception) is a pill a girl takes every day that is extremely effective at preventing pregnancy. It works by releasing a small amount of hormones that fool a girl's brain into thinking she's already pregnant. That way, the brain doesn't stimulate her ovaries to produce an egg. No egg, no pregnancy.

The biggest drawback of birth control pills (or any type of hormonal contraception, be it the pill, the patch, or the ring) are the possible side effects. Those side effects may include: nausea, headaches, breast tenderness, weight gain, weight loss, mood changes, breakthrough bleeding, and missed periods. The two most common complaints about birth control pills are nausea and light bleeding in between periods. But many girls can actually regulate those annoyances by changing the way they take the pill. The more accurate a girl is about taking the pill at the same time each day, the less likely it is that she'll experience breakthrough bleeding. And if your daughter finds the pill makes her nauseous, she can try taking it right before she goes to bed. Any of the side effects your daughter might experience from taking birth control pills may go away after she's been on the pill for a few months. If they don't, she can discuss her symptoms with a health care provider and get switched to another pill that is less likely to produce those symptoms. And if her side effects are that unbearable, she can always stop taking the pill and they will go away within twenty-four hours.

Health wise, the pill is very safe. Although there is a small risk of blood clots, strokes, and heart attacks, these risks are mostly for women over thirty-five who smoke. All in all, it is statistically much less risky to take birth control pills than it is to give birth.

The biggest complaint about the pill versus other methods of hormonal contraception is that some girls find it difficult to remember to take something every day. For this reason, forgetful girls find it helpful to pair taking the pill with something they do each day anyway—like brushing their teeth. Others set an alarm on their cell phone to help them remember. Eventually, it just becomes habit. If a girl can become conditioned to turn off the lights every time she leaves a room, she can remember to take a pill every night before she goes to bed. (It bears mentioning that girls don't have to take the pill at the same time every day. As long as they take the pill every day, when they take it will not impact its effectiveness.)

"The Patch"

PROS: A girl using the patch only has to remember to change it once a week, and the higher levels of estrogen may be more effective at clearing up her skin.

CONS: Girls are more likely to experience breast tenderness and nausea, and some don't like having a visible patch stuck on them. Also, some research suggests the patch is more likely than other forms of contraception to cause blood clots, strokes, and heart attacks.

"The patch" is a small tan patch that sticks on like a Band-Aid, and only has to be changed once a week. A new one is put on every week for three weeks in a row, then a girl takes a week off (and gets her period). The patch delivers hormones similar to those in birth control pills, works the same way as birth control pills, and is very effective at preventing pregnancy. While girls on birth control pills report lighter periods with less cramping, girls on the patch are less likely to experience that beneficial side effect (Lopez et al. 2008). Girls are also more likely to report breast tenderness and nausea when using the patch. As with the pill, any girl who doesn't like the side effects she's having can take it off, and they will go away within a day or so.

"The Ring"

PROS: A girl using the ring only has to remember to take it out every three weeks. While it seems to regulate a girl's period as well as birth control pills, it also seems to be less associated with nausea and mood changes.

CONS: Some girls feel uneasy (at least initially) about inserting it into their vaginas. Also, because the ring is used in the vagina, it may cause vaginal irritation or an increased amount of discharge.

"The ring" (NuvaRing) is a small rubber-like, hormone-filled ring that a girl inserts into the back of her vagina, and leaves there for three weeks. After three weeks she takes it out, spends a week without anything (when she gets her period), and then inserts a new one. Girls who experience bad side effects from birth control pills or the patch may do better on the ring, which seems to cause fewer side effects for many girls. It is also just as effective as the pill and the patch at preventing pregnancy and works the same way.

The biggest drawback of the ring is that some girls feel uncomfortable sticking their fingers into their vaginas to insert it and remove it. Dr. Stuart, an OB-GYN at the University of North Carolina believes that while "there's a lot of initial reluctance to the ring because girls aren't comfortable touching themselves, once they get used to using it, they really like this method of contraception." I would argue that if a girl is too squeamish about sticking her own fingers up her vagina, then maybe she shouldn't be sticking anything else in there either. . . .

Another concern I've heard about the ring comes from young men. They wonder if having sex with a girl who uses the ring is at all harmful to them or their penis—since it will be touching the hormone-filled device. The answer to that question is no. It is not harmful to men in any way, it will not shrink their penis, make them grow boobs, turn them into a woman, or emasculate them in any way. If they're like most guys, they won't even feel the ring during sex.

Since the hormones in the ring are similar to those in birth control pills, it carries similar health benefits of clearing up a girl's skin, and helping to regulate her period. But it also carries the same risks of increasing the chance of blood clots, heart attacks, and strokes.

And just like the pill and the patch, if a girl doesn't like the side effects of the ring, she can just take it out and find a different method of birth control.

WHEN TO CALL THE DOCTOR

Although a girl can stop using the pill, the patch, or the ring if she is having unbearable side effects, it's important that she contact her doctor, tell the doctor she stopped using her method of contraception, and try to find a new one that will work for her.

"The Rod"

PROS: Girls with a contraceptive implant never have to remember to do anything, and because there's no room for human error, it is extremely effective.

CONS: Implantable contraception can be more likely to cause irregular bleeding, depression, and weight gain. Also, some girls don't like the idea of having something implanted in their arm.

"The rod" (Implanon), or implantable contraception, is a small plastic stick about the size of a match that's inserted under the skin in a woman's arm by a doctor. The stick can be in place as long as three years, and it slowly releases hormones to prevent a girl from becoming pregnant. The hormone used in implantable birth control is just a progestin (a hormone that mirrors testosterone—the "male" hormone), not an estrogen (the "female" hormone). In this way, implantable birth control is different from many other forms of hormonal birth control that contain both a progestin and an estrogen (the ring, the patch, and all but one type of birth control pill). Because the hormones are different, implantable birth control has different side effects, health benefits, and health risks. Some of the side effects are the same: nausea and breast tenderness, while others are more pronounced: depression, weight gain, and bleeding between periods. A few side effects are actually the complete opposite: increased acne and hair loss.

If a girl using implantable contraception doesn't like the side effects she can make an appointment with her doctor to have it removed. Once the device is removed, the side effects should go away within twenty-four hours.

The hormones in implantable contraception work in a similar way to those in birth control pills. But as well as tricking a girl's body into thinking she's pregnant, they also thicken the mucus around her cervix, so that even if an egg managed to escape her ovary, the sperm would have a harder time getting to it.

"The Shot"

PROS: A girl using the shot as birth control only has to remember to get it every three months. Again, since there's not much room for human error (assuming a girl gets her shot on time) it is an extremely effective way to prevent pregnancy.

CONS: The shot is more likely to cause depression, weight gain, and irregular bleeding. Also, if a girl doesn't like the side effects of the shot, she has to wait three months for them to go away.

"The shot" (Depo-Provera) is a form of birth control where a girl gets an injection of hormones once every three months. Just like implantable birth control, the shot uses progestin only, so it works the same way, and the side effects are similar (see "The Rod"). The shot is not the most popular form of birth control, and many girls who get one shot never return for a second one. It is the most useful for girls who won't make an effort to remember to use their birth control correctly, don't have a lot of money to spend on birth control, and are able to visit a doctor's office or clinic once every three months.

"The T"/IUD

PROS: Once inserted, it's good for five to ten years, and a girl can forget about it completely. One type of IUD is completely hormone free, and the other type contains a little bit of progesterone and significantly reduces menstrual bleeding.

CONS: Some girls are scared to have it inserted. Also, the type of IUD that has no hormones can significantly increase menstrual flow.

IUDs (intrauterine devices) have come a long way since the Dalkon Shield. An IUD, often called a "T" is a small T-shaped device that's inserted into a girl's uterus by a doctor. It is an extremely effective way to prevent pregnancy. There are two different types of IUDs and they work in different ways. ParaGard, the copper IUD, releases copper into the fluid in the uterus, which creates a toxic environment for sperm (but not for the woman or her reproductive system). Dead sperm equals no pregnancy. The other type of IUD, Mirena, releases a small amount of progesterone each day that prevents pregnancy in the same way as the shot and the implant. The difference is, only a small amount of hormone gets into the blood. Both types of IUDs can be used by a girl of any age, and both are very safe. An IUD won't make a girl more likely to contract an STD, or make one worse if she gets one.

Some girls experience irregular bleeding as a result of using an IUD, and other rarer side effects may include increased cramping or backaches. If a girl doesn't like the IUD, she must make an appointment with a doctor to have it removed. An IUD is an excellent choice for a girl who wants to be able to forget about her birth control method.

Other Options for Preventing Pregnancy

Aside from the methods just mentioned, there are several other ways women can prevent an unwanted pregnancy. The problem with these other methods is that they aren't as effective, they have to be used shortly before sex, they often have more complicated instructions, and they must be inserted into the vagina consistently and correctly in order to be effective. For teens, these methods are usually just too high maintenance. If, however, your daughter is completely opposed to all the other options she may want to ask her doctor about a diaphragm, a cervical cap, or a vaginal sponge.

Things That Don't Prevent Pregnancy (At Least, Not Very Well)

OB-GYN Katharine O'Connell White sees teens regularly and says, "Myths about pregnancy are still shockingly common." Some teens think they can't get pregnant if they have sex standing up; that they won't get pregnant the first time they have sex; and if they've had a lot of unprotected sex and have never gotten pregnant (or gotten someone else pregnant), that they're infertile. I've had girls tell me they didn't think they could get pregnant because they had been anorexic, or because they had done drugs. Quite simply, some teens may have to be told their bodies *are* fertile or that their boys *are* swimmers.

Perhaps the most confusing myths about pregnancy prevention are the ones that are based in some truth. Many teens mistakenly believe a girl can't get pregnant on her period. That myth is based on a form of contraception called "the rhythm method." The rhythm method is used by women to determine the two to three days each month they can get pregnant. Those two to three days occur about twelve days before a girl's *next* period, which theoretically should be about a week after a girl's last period has ended. However, since cycles can be unpredictable, bleeding can be irregular, and semen can live in the vagina for up to seven days, a girl can still get pregnant when she is bleeding (although it may be *less* likely).

REAL-LIFE ADVICE

Next time the issue of pregnancy comes up—whether it's because a friend or neighbor is pregnant, or there is a pregnant character on TV—take the time to clear up some of your child's possible misconceptions. Say, "Despite what you may have heard, a girl can get pregnant the first time she has sex, when she has sex standing up, and when she is on her period. And even if you have unprotected sex a few times and nothing happens, that doesn't mean you're infertile or that a pregnancy won't happen if you do it again—it only means you were lucky enough to dodge some bullets. You may have heard about the 'pull and pray' method, or 'pulling out,' as a way to prevent pregnancy. That is *not* a good form of birth control. But, if you do ever find yourself in the middle of unprotected sex, it is better than nothing."

The other pregnancy myth that has some truth to it is that a girl can't get pregnant if a guy pulls out before he ejaculates. It is true, doing this will decrease the chance of pregnancy, but because pre-ejaculate can contain semen, a girl can still get pregnant if a guy successfully pulls out. And of course there is always the possibility a guy will have the intention of pulling out, but will miscalculate his ejaculation and be just a second too late. Not only does the "pull and pray" method not always work, it can be a difficult thing to do accurately.

Emergency Contraception

Because emergency contraception is taken after sex, many people confuse it with the abortion pill, RU-486. They are *not* the same thing. RU-486 is an abortifacient, meaning that it ends a pregnancy. Emergency contraception *prevents* a girl from becoming pregnant in the first place. It is made up of the same hormones as other hormonal contraceptives, only the doses are higher.

REAL-LIFE ADVICE

Next time you are with your daughter and abortion is being discussed on the radio, on TV, or in conversation, tell her: "A lot of people are misinformed and think taking emergency contraception is the same thing as having an abortion. That is absolutely not true. There is an abortion pill but it's not the same thing as emergency contraception. Even though you take emergency contraception after you have sex, it still *prevents* a potential pregnancy. It can't end one."

Emergency contraception is completely safe, and your daughter should take it if she ever has unprotected sex, has sex after misusing her hormonal method, or when a condom slips off or breaks (and she wasn't using any other form of contraception). If taken within twelve hours, it is 92 percent effective at preventing pregnancy. Although it is more effective if taken sooner, it can be used up to five days after unprotected sex.

The most common side effect associated with emergency contraception is nausea. Girls may want to take an antinausea medication an hour or so beforehand to help them feel less sick. Taking the pills with a full meal may help as well. Other less common side effects of emergency contraception may include throwing up, breast tenderness, irregular bleeding, dizziness, and headaches. Taking emergency contraception may also mess up the timing and length of a girl's next period. It does not, however, have any long-term side effects or cause any health complications.

Anyone seventeen or older can buy emergency contraception over the counter at most pharmacies (Plan B is the most common brand). But since there is so much misinformation about emergency contraception (the abortion misunderstanding), in some parts of the country it may be harder to find. It may be a good idea for you to go ahead and buy a pack just in case. You can either give the pack to your daughter or tell her you have it if she or a friend ever needs to use it.

Taking Your Daughter to the Gynecologist

In order for your daughter to get the most out of a visit to the gynecologist (or any doctor) you should do more than throw her into the car and take her there. Very often, mothers will accompany their daughters to their first appointment with a gynecologist. And while that is a supportive thing to do, you need to make sure that you're still letting your daughter run the show. Parents should "empower their daughters to be wise users of the health care system. It's fine to be there with her for support, but don't take over," says Denniz Zolnoun, OB-GYN at the University of North Carolina at Chapel Hill. The following are the things you should do to give your daughter the skills to fully take advantage of doctors' appointments for the rest of her life.

Make a List

Before going to the gynecologist with your daughter explain what the appointment is like. See if your daughter has any questions: about birth control, her period, her vagina, STDs, or anything else, and tell her to write them down. There may be some questions she doesn't want you to know she has, so tell her that if she has any questions she wants to ask the doctor in private, she can write them down on a separate list or just try to remember them. Either way, get her to start thinking about things she'd like to discuss with the doctor.

PAP SMEARS AND HORMONAL CONTRACEPTION

It's not actually necessary for your daughter to get a pelvic exam until she is sexually active. If she just wants to start taking birth control pills she can visit the gynecologist to talk about her options, but she won't need to get a pelvic exam or a pap smear.

Encourage *Her* to Talk

Don't be an overly pushy parent and talk for your daughter: "Honey, tell the doctor about your menstrual cramps. They were so bad last week we had to take you out of school, and I swear you went through a whole box of super-plus tampons." (Talk about TMI!) Instead, encourage your daughter to speak for herself. If she's not talking, it's fine to prompt her by saying something like, "Were there any questions or concerns you had about your period?" Just don't dominate the visit and start talking over her or putting words in her mouth. Your goal is to empower her to be able to speak for herself and teach her how to communicate with a doctor.

Tell Her to Be a Squeaky Wheel

Not all doctors are the best communicators. And even the ones who are have no way of knowing how much each patient knows about her body or whatever health issue brought her in. Tell your daughter not to worry about asking the doctor a lot of questions. If there is something she doesn't understand, something she wants to know more about, or something the doctor said that wasn't clear, make sure she knows to keep asking until she has all of the information she needs. The doctor's job is to help keep her healthy, and a big part of that job is answering questions.

Step Out

I'm sure you know *everything* about your child's sex life (or lack thereof), but just in case she has some concerns she doesn't want to express in front of you, step out of the room and give her some alone time with the doctor. The only reason not to do this is if your daughter is really scared about the appointment and has specifically asked you ahead of time not to leave her alone. Otherwise, if the doctor doesn't ask you to step out, say to your daughter "I'm going to leave the room for a little bit, is that okay?" And unless she protests, take a seat in the waiting room.

Even if your daughter doesn't have a mother who can take her to the doctor, as a father you can talk with her about being an informed patient and asking a lot of questions (although, during the actual appointment I would stay in the waiting room and leaf through *Pregnancy Today*). And even if you have a son (who obviously doesn't need to see a gyno), you can still teach him about how to take full advantage of a doctor's appointment. That is a skill that everyone can use to stay healthy in any aspect of their lives.

CONTRACEPTION CHEAT SHEET

Below is a summary of the things you should tell your daughter about contraception.

1. Many of the side effects of contraception are greatly exaggerated. As many women lose weight on the pill as gain; the pill doesn't cause cancer; and if you feel like the pill you're taking is affecting your mood, your stomach, your head, your period, or anything else, there are sixty-eight other kinds to try. You can also go on another method all together.
2. If you don't want to have to remember to take a pill every day, there's a patch you only change once a week, a ring you change every month, a shot you get every three months, or an implant that will last for three years.
3. There are two new types of IUDs that are both completely safe and very effective, and once you get one inserted, you'll never have to think about birth control.
4. Taking emergency contraception is not the same as having an abortion. Emergency contraception prevents a pregnancy from happening, it doesn't end one. Anyone over seventeen can now buy emergency contraception at most pharmacies.

And these are the things you should remember yourself:

1. There are many different contraceptive options: the pill, the patch, the ring, the implant, the shot, the IUD, and

more. Work with your daughter and her doctor to find one that is best suited for her.

2. Sex can be unexpected. Birth control can mess up. It might be a good idea to keep some emergency contraception in the house.
3. You are your daughter's access to the health care system, not your daughter's stand-in. While you should take the initiative to make appointments and accompany your daughter to them, don't take over. Let her do the talking.
4. Teach your children—sons or daughters—to be informed patients. Tell them to write down any questions they have ahead of time and make sure that during the appointment their doctor adequately addresses their concerns.

Chapter Eight WHAT GIRLS NEED TO KNOW

The thing that strikes me as odd is how many young women have it all figured out—they're bold, beautiful, smart, and then as soon as they get in bed they lose their voice.

–Linda Brown, MPH, health education consultant, South Carolina State Health Department

The average age a girl starts having sex is eighteen. But many women don't have their first orgasm until some time in their twenties. Other women will tell you they didn't really like sex until they were in their thirties. For many young women, sex is a guy thing, and they're just along for the ride. But in order for girls to be sexually healthy and make good decisions, they need to be put in the driver's seat when it comes to their sex life. This chapter is about the assumptions, misunderstandings, and stereotypes that make girls insecure about sex and relationships.

Maybe you're reading this thinking: not my daughter, she's not insecure; she'll never need help asserting herself. She's so smart, or beautiful, or confident, or all of those things. But how many amazing women do you know who were never able to parlay their intelligence and confidence into good romantic decisions? There's nothing like sex and love to make a smart girl stupid. No matter how amazing or confident your daughter may be, she still needs empowerment when it comes to love and sex.

The "Truth" about Sex

Sex is something people *love* to talk about. Teens get flooded with all sorts of ideas about how sex affects a relationship, a crush, and their relationships with friends. Especially when a girl is a virgin, she has no way of knowing if those ideas are true or not. And even when a girl becomes sexually active it might take her a while to sort out fact from fiction. The following are a few misunderstandings many young women have about sex and what you can say to clear them up.

Sex Will Get a Guy or Keep Him Interested

Some girls believe the only thing they have to offer a guy is sex. They think that if they want a chance with a guy who's not immediately interested, their best bet is to hook up with him. Other girls worry that if they don't have sex with a guy they've been dating for a while (especially a guy who's had sex before), he'll leave. They hear, "sex is a way for two people to build intimacy in a relationship" and interpret that to mean, "Sex can make a guy like you."

Convince your daughter that the way to a man's heart is not through his zipper. Tell her, "Having sex with a guy is not going to make him change the way he feels about you or create an intimate bond that's not already there. When you have sex with a guy, make sure you're happy with the relationship you have before you sleep with him, and that you're not expecting a better relationship to surface afterward."

TMI WARNING

While you may want to share your own experiences with your children and help them learn from your mistakes, some things about your past may be best left out. Like that weird "relationship" you had with the TA that consisted of you sleeping with him after class. Or the crazy girl who insisted you would fall in love with her if you let her spend the night with you. If it involves any sort of details about you having sex, your daughter doesn't want to know.

Sex Will Make Me Feel Wanted

Some girls hook up because they're craving attention or searching for validation that they're attractive. And what's most difficult about getting your daughter to avoid this habit is that it's not usually a conscious thought process. Most girls don't actively think, "I feel ugly and unlovable so I'm going to hook up with someone." But if they were to analyze the motivation behind their sexual decisions afterward, many could tell you they've had sex for the temporary gratification of feeling wanted. Of course, that's a very fleeting solution to a much bigger problem of low self-esteem.

Hopefully, throughout your daughter's life you've instilled a sense of self-worth, value, and respect. And if you notice she doesn't feel those things, do everything you can to boost her confidence (see Chapter 1). But regardless of how positive you believe your daughter's self-image is, it is always a good idea to tell her sex should never be used as a way for her to feel wanted and attractive. She should know that approach always flops, and in the long run it will only make her feel badly about herself.

I Should Have Sex to Be Like Everyone Else

Stereotypically, we think of guys as the ones who are motivated to have sex by the desire to impress or bond with their friends. But if your daughter is part of a sexually experienced crowd, the pressure for her can be just as great. In a national survey, 44 percent of teen girls said their friends influenced their decision about becoming sexually active (Kaiser Family Foundation and *Seventeen* 2000). If all of your daughter's friends are sitting around talking about sex, she probably doesn't want to be "the prude" who has nothing to add.

It's always a good idea to encourage your children to think for themselves and not just go with the crowd. But for this particular situation, I'd also explain that a lot of teens are full of it when it comes to sex. Tell her, "Sometimes your friends might try to play it cool, and act like sex is no big deal. But on the inside they're probably totally freaked out about it." Also tell her that anyone who feels okay about her own decision to have sex won't be overly preoccupied with what her friends are doing. And let your daughter know that no one who's a good friend will like her any less for being sexually inexperienced.

REAL-LIFE ADVICE

If you think your daughter is running with a fast crowd, give her this advice: "You don't have to be sexually experienced to be able to gossip about sex. You can ask about your friends' experiences, talk with them about boys they like, or tell them about something you read online. You don't have to have sex too just to not feel left out."

Boys Aren't Assholes

Teens, adults, TV shows, self-help books, and ad campaigns just can't get enough of this whole "guys only want sex" bit. Girls grow up hearing about how guys hate relationships and are only out for "one thing." They are warned: "be careful of lying guys who will use you for sex." They're cautioned against guys who say "I love you" just because they want to get laid. But not only are these stereotypes completely played out, they're just not true.

First of all, I can't say I've ever heard of a guy lying about his intentions in order to sleep with a girl. This is not to say that some young men aren't interested in casual sex, but more often than not, that's pretty apparent. More importantly, however, is the point that the vast majority of guys aren't just out for sex. They have feelings, get crushes, are interested in relationships, and care about more than just getting off. Yes, guys are people too.

When I give lectures to coed audiences it always goes down the same way. In the big group guys are quick to hoot and holler about anything sexual, but afterward they come up to me one-on-one, and sing a different tune. They don't ask me how to get a girl in bed; they ask things like: "I really like a girl in my class but don't know how to approach her," or "I have a crush on my friend and I want to turn our friendship into something more." Despite what your daughter has likely been told, teenage guys don't just like girls because they like sex, they like girls because they enjoy girls' company. Many young men find comfort in female companionship, and find it easier to talk with girls about things they would never feel comfortable discussing with their guy friends. And although many people think of relationships as "a girl thing," studies show that young men have a much more difficult time coping when a relationship ends. Studies also show that down the road, married men are happier than married women—something one might not expect, given the whole ball-and-chain stereotype.

As an adult, this may all be obvious information to you, but are these the types of things you say about guys in front of your daughter? That they enjoy relationships and female companionship? Very likely, the fact that guys have feelings and actually *enjoy* relationships will hit her like a brick wall: "Holy Crap! You mean guys want more than just booty!"

NEWSFLASH TO YOUR DAUGHTER

Many girls are also shocked to find out that guys have fears and insecurities about sex too. While it's true that many young men want to have sex, they worry about their performance, the size of their penis, and what the girl is going to think about their moves. Your daughter should know: Sex isn't easy for them either.

Why Your Daughter Needs to Know Boys Aren't Assholes

The problem with the "guys are assholes" message is that it completely backfires. While the guys who will say "I love you" in order to get laid may be few and far between, what's very common are the girls who have sex because they think it's the only way to make a guy happy. When the message "all guys want is sex" is drilled into girls' heads, instead of preventing sex, it can actually encourage it. If a girl really likes a guy, and she thinks the only thing he wants is sex, then it's no mystery what she's going to do to get him.

This message also backfires in that it encourages girls to say that all they want is sex as well. No one wants to be a sucker. Why would girls want to chase after a guy for a relationship he doesn't want? It's much easier for girls to say, "All you want is sex? Fine. That's all I want too." Many girls think it's just more realistic to lower their expectation for the type of relationship they can have—which in my opinion, is a contributing factor to the "hookup culture" on college campuses. Although I do think the "hookup culture" phenomenon is part truth, part media hype, I also think many girls believe their best bet is to toughen up and have sex "like a guy" (without any emotional commitment). That way, it keeps them from being vulnerable—a guy can't screw you if you screw him first.

Now, imagine that we were able to convince all young women that guys were decent human beings who want more than "just one thing." Suppose girls were taught that guys like relationships and that they value intelligence, a sense of humor, and a kind soul. For one, romantic relationships would seem much more obtainable and appealing. But secondly, girls would have an easier time learning to value those traits in themselves. When we tell girls that guys only want them for their vaginas, they get the message that their value lies solely within their sexuality. Wonder why so many teen girls seem overly consumed with their bodies, clothing, and makeup? Because we inadvertently support the notion that a girl's biggest asset is her sex appeal. If girls were raised hearing "what guys want is a girl who's ambitious," then to impress a guy, they would be hitting their books, not jumping into the sack.

What you tell your daughter about the opposite sex matters. It affects both how she will approach romantic relationships and what she will value in herself. Illuminating the fact that guys are real people with real emotions makes them less intimidating and makes it easier for girls to know what they should expect out of a relationship. If you let your daughter believe that guys are assholes, how can you insist she have standards for the type of guys she dates? Why not date losers—if all guys are jerks anyway.

REAL-LIFE ADVICE

This might be the most powerful coming from Dad. Although with many topics in this book I'd advise you to leave yourself out of it, this is a good place for you to tell a story about yourself. Dad, what was something you did to impress a girl? Tell your daughter: "The way guys are portrayed on TV is awful. They're made out to be these jerks who would do anything to get in a girl's pants. But the vast majority of guys aren't like that. They're totally intimidated by girls they like and do all sorts of stupid things to impress them. Many guys want to have a girlfriend. They want a girl they can hang out with, joke around with, and talk to, not just someone to have sex with. There are plenty of great guys out there who will make fantastic boyfriends, so never settle for a guy that treats you badly or isn't giving you everything you want, because he isn't worth your time."

Sex is Supposed to Be Good

Last summer I spent a few days staying with the teenage daughter of a family friend. One night we ordered pizzas and had her friends over for a sex talk. At first, all of the girls who had had sex were joking around about different positions, how they lost their virginity, and all the crazy places they had done it. Then I asked them if they had orgasms when they had sex. The room got quiet. I asked if they enjoyed sex, and if it actually felt good. I got some mumbles and a lot of "sorta," "maybe," "kinda." Somehow, they weren't aware that sex should be physically pleasurable for them too. Even though they were sexually active, their own enjoyment wasn't something that factored into the equation.

Of all the things that girls are told about sex, very few are told that they're supposed to like it. Many parents are afraid if they let girls in on the secret that sex *can* be amazing they'll raise little nymphos. So instead, when they talk to girls about sex they stick to the "safe" messages: "You could really regret having sex," "Sex can make you feel used," "Sex means you have to worry about STDs and pregnancy." Basically, sex sucks.

But here's the problem with raising girls to think so negatively about sex: If they expect sex to be bad, how are they supposed to recognize when they are having sex in a bad situation with an unsupportive partner? They'll just think: "I guess sex is supposed to be lame when you're a girl." If instead you tell your daughter that in the right situation sex is wonderful, then when she's in a situation where sex obviously wouldn't be wonderful she'll know not to do it. Making clear to your daughter that sex should be pleasurable will only help her make better choices about when to have sex.

A Girl's Sexual Desire Is Important

Young women need to understand that girls have sexual desires and that those desires matter. It's not just guys who want sex; girls want sex too. Yes, girls get horny (but don't phrase it that way to your daughter). The problem with young women not recognizing their own sexual desire is that it means every time they have sex it's for a guy, because sex was something *he* wanted to do. And that sets them up to feel victimized because it means they are having sex for someone else instead of for themselves.

Girls need to be reminded of the importance of their sexual desires because they're so bombarded with messages about guys' desires. It's the myth of the holy hard-on: guys get really turned on because they get boners. For that reason, if you start to hook up with a guy, you can't stop or he'll get blue balls. And if a guy does something sexual to you, it's only fair that you do it back to him. Guys have sexual desires that *matter*!

Your daughter must know that her sexual desires matter too and that her sexual pleasure is just as important as a guy's. If she doesn't, how can you expect her to demand that a guy use a condom if she's thinking that his physical enjoyment is more important than her own? If she's out of her comfort zone, how can you expect her to get up and leave if she thinks it's unfair to abandon a guy once he's turned on? If you want your daughter to eventually have an enjoyable sex life, how can she do that if she's always placing what feels good for a guy over what feels good for her? Part of helping your daughter have a healthy sex life means helping her understand that her desires count. In order to make the best choices about sex and their sexual health, young women need to be sexually empowered. And part of that empowerment means making them understand that sex is theirs to enjoy.

Getting Girls to Stand Up for Themselves in Bed

Sex isn't just "a guy thing." Girls need to know it's something that's under their control, and they have power in the bedroom too. They need to be active players with opinions, boundaries, and desires. They shouldn't be getting into sexual situations by going with the flow, shrugging their shoulders and saying, "I don't know. I guess I'm okay with this."

Part of getting girls to set clear boundaries is getting them to figure out ahead of time what those boundaries are. Encourage your daughter to think about the types of situations where she thinks sex is a good idea and it would be most enjoyable. Have her think about the following: What types of sex acts—in which situations—convey respect for both her and her partner? What does it take for her to feel respected by a partner? What does it take for her to feel like she is respecting herself? How can she make sure that a sexual situation is meeting her needs as well as his?

Questions to Help Your Daughter Define Her Sexual Boundaries

- Do you think sex is a good idea when you're drunk or high?
- Do you think it's a good idea to have sex with a guy because he really wants to?
- Would you feel comfortable having oral sex with a guy when you weren't in a relationship with him? Would you feel good about that the next day? The next week?
- What types of sex acts do you enjoy? (Don't answer that out loud!)
- If you don't feel respected in a sexual situation would you get up and leave?
- If you wanted to leave a situation, what would you say? (Perhaps suggest your daughter practice by saying something to you.)
- If a friend's crush was coming on to you, do you think it would be okay to hook up with him?
- What would you do if a guy didn't want to use a condom?

Girls should go into sexual situations with a definite sense of what's okay and what isn't. Then, they need to be able to assert their needs. Some girls worry that if they have an opinion that's different from their guy's, he will lose interest. They worry about not having sex when a guy wants to, not having oral sex with a guy whose friends are all getting BJs, or asking to use a condom when they know it will reduce a guy's physical pleasure. But beyond the fact that a girl owes it to herself to respect her own needs, she needs to be convinced that her boundaries will not make a guy like her any less.

REAL-LIFE ADVICE

When talking to your daughter about sexual boundaries, be sure to tell her: "It's not cute to be passive when it comes to sex. Guys have more respect for girls who are in control, know if they want to have sex or not, and stick to their guns. If a guy likes you, he likes you, and any decision you make either way isn't going to change that. Form an opinion. Stick with it. And know it won't change a guy's true feelings."

Make clear to your daughter: if a guy likes her, the fact that she's respecting her needs will only make him like and respect her more. And if a guy doesn't like her, there is nothing she can do to change that. Having sex with him, going down on him, or letting him have sex with her without a condom will not change his feelings.

Help her believe this by flipping the situation around. What if she really liked a guy she was dating and wanted to have sex but he wasn't ready (and this may happen to her one day). Would she stop having feelings for him? Would she say, "forget you" and move on to someone else? No, she would respect his needs. And as previously noted, guys are people too, and their minds work the same way.

Examining "Slut"

Your daughter will hear, be victimized by, and maybe even perpetuate sexual stereotypes. That is unavoidable. Realistically, it's impossible to completely rid our culture of them. Your best bet as a parent is to teach your kids to be aware of them, reject them, and do their best not to judge others by these outdated ideas.

The most prevalent stereotype your kids will encounter is the idea that a girl who has a lot of sex is a slut. These days, the definition of a slut has gotten a little looser. Maybe a girl hasn't slept with that many people, but she slept with a guy your daughter liked: "that slut face!" Or an ex-boyfriend: "the little slut bag." But no matter how the term is used, it's supporting the idea that a girl being sexual is pitiful, wrong, or dirty.

Of course, your daughter would never want to be called a slut, but the threat of the slut idea goes much deeper than that. If girls are afraid of someone thinking they're slutty, than they're probably not going to feel that comfortable carrying condoms. If girls don't believe they should be having premeditated thoughts about sex, then how are they supposed to plan ahead and decide when sex is okay and when it isn't. And if they can't demand that their sexual pleasure matters too (because it sounds too sexually aggressive), how can they stand up for themselves in the bedroom?

Since you probably won't be able to erase the idea of a "slut" from your daughter's head, help her examine what she really thinks it means. Help her differentiate between so-called "slutty behaviors" and a girl simply thinking about, being prepared for, and engaging in sex. Ask her: "Is being prepared and responsible slutty? Is it slutty to stand up for yourself? Is it slutty to think that you're as important as a guy?" Guide her to the conclusion that it's not slutty to be sexually prepared, enjoy sex, have definite opinions about sex, or be a sexually active woman. When a girl is respecting herself and her needs, she's not being a slut; she's taking control of her sexuality.

I'm not saying that the term or idea of a "slut" is okay, but since it's so prevalent in our society, like it or not, it's something you need to address head on. And that means not simply telling her the idea is wrong, but helping her have a firm grasp on which sexual behaviors she thinks are okay and which sexual behaviors she thinks aren't.

REAL-LIFE ADVICE

Chances are, one day you'll hear your son or daughter call someone a slut. Take that opportunity and call him or her on it: "What is a slut?" "Can a guy be a slut—and what would that look like?" "Would you want someone calling you a slut because you had sex? Is that fair?" Explain to your kids: "The problem with using the word 'slut' is that it doesn't just insult the girl you've used it about, it perpetuates that stereotype for all women. I hope you know that girls can have sex, prepare for sex, and enjoy sex and that doesn't mean they're slutty. There is nothing slutty about being ready for sex by carrying a condom or thinking ahead of time about whether or not you think sex is a good idea."

WHAT TO TELL YOUR DAUGHTERS CHEAT SHEET

Below is a summary of the topics you should talk about with your daughters.

1. Having sex with a guy will not make him like you if he doesn't already. It's also not going to add intimacy to a relationship that doesn't have any intimacy in the first place.
2. It's never a good idea to have sex for a self-esteem boost or to feel attractive. In the end, that will only make you feel worse.
3. Not everyone is having sex, and you don't have to either. You can still talk with your sexually active friends about their experiences, or share your thoughts about your own—even if those experiences don't include intercourse.
4. Guys want more than just sex. They are people too. They enjoy a girl's company, her intelligence, kindness, and sense of humor, and they enjoy relationships. They also have their own concerns in the sex department. Sex isn't a breeze for them either.
5. You probably hear a lot about how important a guy's sexual satisfaction is, but yours is every bit as important. Your sexual desires carry just as much weight as his.
6. What types of sex acts—in which situations—convey respect for both you and your partner? What does it take for you to feel respected by a partner? What does it take for you to feel like you're respecting yourself? Figure out your sexual boundaries and stick to them. And know that sticking to your guns isn't going to make your partner like you any less.
7. First of all, you're not helping anyone when you use the term "slut." Second of all, there is nothing "slutty" about thinking about sex, being prepared for it, and expressing your sexual needs.

Chapter Nine
WHAT BOYS NEED TO KNOW

Having two older brothers I had learned all the important facts before the age of ten:

1. *Girls piss out of their assholes,*
2. *A man gets a woman pregnant by peeing on her, and*
3. *(My personal favorite) my sisters–who are eleven months apart—were really twins, but one wasn't ready to come out right away.*

—Steve, age fifty-five

Throughout this entire book, as I've said "talk with your kids about sex," I don't just mean "talk to your daughters." You have to talk to your sons too. With as little quality information as young women receive about sex, young men get even less. Whenever I talk on college campuses—even if the posters are geared toward girls—guys usually make up at least half my audience. And the ones who come aren't there just to snicker at a girl talking about genitalia; they come with thoughtful questions about relationships, sex, and their bodies. As one guy put it, "You don't understand, *no one* talks to us about sex." Clearly, this is something young people internalize because 61 percent of teens say that boys receive the message that sex and pregnancy aren't a big deal (The National Campaign to Prevent Teen and Unplanned Pregnancy 2007).

Boys need to know that sex *is* a big deal and that they're not giant wusses for thinking so. Even though they aren't the ones who get pregnant, they still need to make thoughtful and responsible choices about sex. Because guys are more physically intimidating, they need to learn to always respect a girl's boundaries, always ask for consent, and know when playful behavior is crossing the line. In a society that expects men to be the bad guys—always trying to trick women into sex and get out of emotional commitments—parents need to tell their sons, "that's not the way real men behave." This chapter is about the topics to discuss with your son, to make sure he approaches sex and relationships in a healthy, safe, and thoughtful way.

Allowing Boys to Be Human

For the most part, the type of conversation that boys have about sex and relationships begins and ends at "Dude, where's your condom?" Culturally speaking, we don't talk with them about any concerns they may have about sex, or how to say "no." (It's just assumed they're trying to get laid at all costs.) Guys aren't encouraged to show a lot of emotion or talk about their feelings. And they're told they won't enjoy being in relationships—other than the fact that a relationship may lead to sex. But your son needs to know these things aren't true. Having trepidations about sex, wanting to make good decisions, and falling in love are not "girl" desires, they're human desires. Help your son break out of the narrow definition of masculinity carved around him by telling him what sex and relationships are *really* like for guys.

Guys Can Say "No" to Sex

You may think of girls as the ones who feel pressure when it comes to sex, but guys are actually *more* likely to report feeling pressured into it. According to a national survey of over 500 teens, 83 percent of guys said that teens face pressure when it comes to sex. When compared to girls, guys felt more pressure to have sex by a certain age, and they were twice as likely to say, "Sex is expected in a relationship" (Kaiser Family Foundation and *Seventeen* 2000).

The message that guys should be sexually experienced is one that sinks in early. In a study of teenage boys aged twelve to nineteen, almost a quarter said they would feel embarrassed to admit they were virgins (The National Campaign to Prevent Teen and Unplanned Pregnancy 2002). And surprisingly, the younger boys surveyed were actually more likely to think being a virgin was embarrassing. Your son needs to know that having sex is a big physical and emotional responsibility, and not one he should necessarily feel ready to take on. He should also know that not all the "cool kids" are doing it, and that he's not obligated to have sex just because he's a guy. There is nothing wrong with waiting, and nothing wrong with being a virgin.

REAL-LIFE ADVICE
Convince your son that having sex is a matter of personal choice, the right circumstances, and that becoming sexually active should have nothing to do with his friends. Say, "If a friend ever makes fun of you for not having sex, that's probably just his insecurities talking. Maybe the guy had sex and the girl told him he sucked at it. Maybe he regrets letting himself get peer-pressured into having sex. Or maybe he's worried about his own inexperience. Either way, anyone who is secure with his own sexual choices wouldn't make fun of yours."

Guys Don't *Have* to Want Sex

Not only is it okay for guys not to have sex, it's okay for them to be intimidated by it. A guy confided in me once that the first time he touched a vagina it was the scariest thing he'd ever felt. Not only was he not turned on, he was terrified. Getting acquainted with the other gender's genitalia can be frightening, for guys as well as girls. And even once it's familiar, performing the actual act of sex is really intimidating for many young men: they have to achieve an erection, maintain an erection, and not get too excited too quickly.

Although I don't think as a parent it's necessarily your job to ease your son's fears about sexual performance, I do think you should clearly tell him that despite what they may act like, nearly all young men are a little freaked out and unsure about sex. Your son should know there is nothing unmanly about not wanting to have sex in every situation where it's a possibility. Young men aren't dogs sitting under the table waiting for whatever scraps get thrown in their general direction. Guys are people too, and they should think carefully about their sexual choices—not just assume that sex is always something they want.

Guys Enjoy Relationships

It may be necessary to make the seemingly obvious statement to your son that it's normal for men to enjoy relationships and develop feelings for someone. Be sure he knows that he doesn't need to put up a front like he doesn't care about girls, and that it's not manly to be emotionally distant and keep the girls he dates at arm's length. As he gets older and starts having relationships, encourage him to be a considerate and attentive boyfriend. (And if his friends give him crap for being "whipped," tell him they're just jealous.) Make sure he understands it's normal to get crushes and fall in love, and that it's okay for men to have and show their feelings.

REAL-LIFE ADVICE

If it's an option, this may be a topic that dads should bring up with their sons. Sons look up to their fathers as their male role model, and if Dad is admitting it's not manly to always be after sex, it must be true. Tell your teen: "Anyone who tells you they're not a little scared to have sex is totally full of it and just trying to act macho. Some guys will act like they're completely ready for sex and that there's something wrong with you if you aren't always thinking about it. There's nothing embarrassing about not wanting to have sex, and it's normal to be uneasy and want to wait until you're truly ready."

You can encourage your son to be in touch with his feelings and talk about his emotions by nurturing that trait throughout his entire life. Support him when he's upset and let him know it's okay to cry. Make sure he understands that it's normal to feel sad, and help him distinguish feeling upset from feeling angry (a favor his future girlfriends will thank you for profusely.) If he's scared to do something, don't go over the top pushing him to be brave and do it anyway; let him know it's okay to be cautious. And when you see portrayals of the typical stoic-ass-of-a-man in the media, remind your son that although that's what some guys may act like on the outside, they're feeling a lot more on the inside.

Teach Your Son to Take Contraception and Pregnancy Seriously

A survey conducted in 2000 by The National Campaign to Prevent Teen and Unplanned Pregnancy showed that 49 percent of teens believe a girl has the most influence over whether or not a condom is used, 13 percent said a boy had the most influence, and 35 percent said it was equal. From these stats, we can assume that teens are viewing contraception as a woman's responsibility. But guys shouldn't be sitting around twiddling their thumbs waiting for girls to tell them to use condoms.

Even though he can't get pregnant, your son should understand that the burden to protect a girl from an unplanned pregnancy falls equally as hard on him. Unplanned pregnancies are no picnic for guys either. If he *does* get a girl pregnant, he doesn't get the final say about what she does with that pregnancy. Whether he is in favor of abortion or not, she may have one. And no matter how ready he feels to be a father, or how much he wants to pay thousands of dollars in child support each year, she is the one who will decide if she wants to have the baby. So even though a baby isn't going to be popping out of your son, he still needs to realize that being on the other side of an unplanned pregnancy is a big deal. And he owes it to both himself and his partner to prevent it from happening.

All pregnancy issues aside, guys get STDs. And that, in and of itself, should make your son want to use a condom. Maybe it will reduce his enjoyment of sex, or maybe it will feel awkward to put on, but he needs to remember that the prospect of contracting an STD is much worse. (For more about counteracting negative feelings about condoms refer back to Chapter 6.)

When talking to your son about condom use, I would frame it this way: it is his penis, and he needs to take the responsibility to make sure it's in a condom. He is responsible for putting on his own jacket before walking out into the cold. He is responsible for making sure he packs a bathing suit before going to a pool. And he is the one who needs to make sure his penis is tucked into a condom before he has sex. It is not a girl's job to remind him or convince him to use one. Using a condom is a guy's only way to share some of the responsibility of contraception, and it is the best way to help prevent the spread of STDs. If he's big boy enough to have sex, he's big boy enough to do so while wearing a condom.

Teach Your Son How to Approach Sex

It's a message that girls get all the time: think about sex before you do it. "Make sure it's not too soon," we tell them, "make sure it's the right person," "make sure you won't regret it." But the message to approach sex cautiously is one that guys need to hear too. Boys who have sex in situations they shouldn't don't feel any better about it than girls.

Tell your son that sex is a big deal—and not just the first time, but every time. It can bring up lots of emotions, fears, and responsibilities—ones that aren't solved by using a condom. A guy needs to make sure sex is something he's prepared to deal with physically and emotionally, and that he thinks it's appropriate for the relationship he is in. When deciding whether or not sex is a good idea, he needs to make sure that he wants to do it for the right reasons. Those reasons being along the lines of "I feel truly ready, and this is something I want to do," not "well, why not?" Boys are not being told enough to think consciously and carefully about their sexual choices—a fact that's only adding to guys thinking they *should* be sexually active, and jump at every opportunity to have sex.

Part of teaching your son about making conscious sexual choices means teaching him to make choices based on his partner's well-being as well as his own. Through media messages and locker room banter, some guys get conditioned to see sex as a "been there," "done that" type of experience rather than a loving act between two people. Your mission, should you choose to accept it, is to challenge that view. Convince your son that it's wrong to view sex as a game or a conquest. You've always taught your kids to treat others the way they would like to be treated, and sex is no exception. Explain that a guy should have sex because he wants to share an intimate act with a person he respects. Having sex with a different motivation (i.e., just to "do" someone or to be able to brag to friends), is not only disrespectful to his partner, it's disrespectful to himself because it means acting in a way that should go against his moral code. Put simply: he's better than that.

If your son is expressing an "it's cool to score with girls" attitude, challenge him on it. Ask him: "It's cool because your friends say it is?" (So you're not man enough to form your own opinions?) "It's cool because girls will think more of you if you're experienced?" (Doubt that's the case.) "It's cool because that's the way guys act in movies?" (Well, guess what, they're acting—that's not real life.) The more you challenge your son to think about the attitudes he has about sex, the easier it will be for him to see though the BS messages about the ways guys "should" approach intimate relationships and sexuality.

GOOD IDEA/BAD IDEA

Here's a little game you might want to play with your son next time you're alone together. Use this to start a conversation about when it's appropriate to have sex. (See the "correct" answers below.)

1. Having sex because the girl you're dating wants to . . . good idea/bad idea?
2. Having sex because you're the last virgin in your group of friends . . . good idea/bad idea?
3. Having sex because you and your partner are ready to physically take your relationship to the next level . . . good idea/bad idea?
4. Having sex so that you have something cool to tell your friends . . . good idea/bad idea?
5. Having sex because you have thought about it and know it's something you are ready to do . . . good idea/bad idea.

ANSWERS:

1. **Bad idea.** Just because a girl wants to have sex doesn't mean you or your relationship is necessarily ready for it. Besides, just because she's a girl it doesn't necessarily mean she wants to have sex for the right reasons.
2. **Bad idea.** There is nothing wrong with being a virgin, and anyone who would make fun of you for it is clearly insecure about his own sexual choices.
3. **Possibly a good idea.** Sex should be something you decide to do with a partner because you want to share that experience with someone you care about.
4. **Bad idea**. Having sex just to impress your friends is a good way to rack up regrets because you're not doing it as a result of your own desires.

5. **Possibly a good idea**. You should decide to have sex because it's something *you* want to do, not because a girl, your friends, or anything else pressures you into it.

Explain Your Son's Responsibilities to Women and in Relationships

I'm not trying to man-hate with this section, but we have to be honest about the fact that the majority of sexual assault assailants and physical abusers are men. I also think we have to be honest about the fact that, for the most part, men aren't born with violent tendencies toward women; they learn them. As the parent of a young man, there's a lot you can do to ensure that your son always treats women (or men for that matter) with kindness and respect. Not just so that he won't become abusive, but so that he'll be a sweet and loving partner. Consider this the new and improved "be a gentleman" talk:

A Girl Never Owes You Sex

Many date rape situations may stem from a guy thinking, for one reason or another, that a girl owes him sex. Guys need to know that just because a girl went up to his room, started to hook up with him, is dressed a certain way, or has a certain reputation, she never "owes" a guy sex. Sex should always be a mutual decision, and something that both people *want* to be doing. A guy shouldn't want to have sex with a girl who's doing it just because she thinks she "owes it to him" anyway.

The Burden Is on You to Ask for Consent

Because a guy is likely physically stronger than the girl he is dating, the burden to ask for sexual consent falls on him. A guy should never just assume that what he's doing is okay, he should always check in and ask. He should know how to look for physical cues as well as verbal cues that a girl is getting uncomfortable.

If she suddenly stops kissing him back, or becomes stiff and unresponsive, he needs to stop all physical action. Very often, young adults end up in sexual situations after they have been drinking. Guys must understand that a girl can't give consent to have sex if she is drunk, high, or passing out.

Your Desire Should Never Come at the Expense of Hurting Someone Else

The urge to have sex can be really strong for young men. There's nothing wrong with that. What is wrong is when that urge is used as an excuse for acting physically or emotionally irresponsible. Whether it's taking off a condom to get more sensation, or having sex with a good friend's ex, it's never okay for a guy to let his little head speak louder than his big one.

TMI WARNING

Dear Fathers, you should make every effort to relate to your son, and talk to him in a way that's accessible. But don't go over the top by showing him "horny Dad," and saying things like, "With all that hot ass running around your school, you may want to screw so bad that you're tempted to make irresponsible choices."

Your Girlfriend Is Not Your Property

The feeling of falling in love for the first time can be overwhelming for anyone. It's only natural for a guy to feel protective of a girl he cares about and want to be around her a lot. But guys need to know that those sentiments can go too far. It's never okay for a guy to try to control how a girl dresses, what she does, or who her friends are. If he's truly worried about her safety, that's one thing, but if it's an issue of "I don't want other guys looking at you," "I don't want you to go out dancing," or "I don't want you to hang out with your guy friends unless I'm there," those demands aren't okay. A boyfriend's job isn't to tell his girlfriend what she can and cannot do.

Never Use Your Physical Strength to Harm

Many guys don't understand that girls can be intimidated by a man's strength (even if only subconsciously). Most guys know it's wrong to hit a girl they're dating, but it's more complicated than that. Guys should never threaten a girl, get violent around her, or throw anything in her general direction. Beyond that, a guy may not even be able to horse around with a girl the same way he can with his guy friends. While wrestling around and throwing a few punches with the guys may be accepted behavior in a friendship, doing that to a girl could really scare her because she probably isn't as strong.

Abuse Is More Than Just Physical

Having a healthy relationship is more than two people not hitting each other. Guys need to know that it's never okay for them to threaten, belittle, or humiliate their girlfriend. That counts as abuse too. They also need to know that that type of abuse is something a girl can just as easily do to a guy. Respect and kindness is a two-way street, and not only should guys give it in a relationship, they should make sure they're receiving it too.

There's most certainly a woman in your family that your son loves and respects. As a golden rule, teach him to treat every woman he has a romantic relationship with the way he would want his mother/sister/aunt/cousin/grandmother to be treated. The girls he dates *are* somebody's sister, someone's best friend, and one day possibly someone's mother and grandmother as well.

WHAT TO TELL YOUR SONS CHEAT SHEET

Below is a summary of the topics you should talk about with your sons.

1. Though some guys may act like it, no one wants sex 100 percent of the time. That's okay and that's normal. It's also normal to find sex intimidating.
2. Don't worry about what other guys may be saying about sex. If they make fun of you for not having sex, it's only because they're insecure with their own choices.
3. It's normal for guys to want relationships and have girlfriends. Having a girlfriend and being good to her doesn't mean you're "whipped."
4. Sex is a big deal, and it's something you should think about carefully.
5. It's not a girl's responsibility to tell you to use a condom. You need to take the initiative to protect the girl you're sleeping with from an unplanned pregnancy, and protect both of you from STDs.
6. No matter what, a girl never owes you sex. It's up to you to continue checking in with a girl you're being intimate with, and make sure you have her consent. Never just assume that it's okay to have sex if she hasn't told you it is.
7. There's a lot to learn the first time you're in a serious relationship. Your job as a boyfriend is never to tell your girlfriend what to do, what to wear, or dictate whom she hangs out with. It's your job to treat her with kindness and respect, never physically hurt her, say nasty things to her, threaten her, try to humiliate her, or try to intimidate her. And make sure that she is just as respectful to you.

Chapter Ten SEXUAL EMERGENCIES

Even your most perfect teen could get into a crisis situation. The thing to remember is that crises aren't the worst thing in the world—though they may feel like it at the time. Getting through one can bring you closer to your child and help your relationship grow.

—Louise Miller Lavin, psychiatric clinical nurse specialist and licensed professional clinical counselor

You do all you can to prepare your children for the sexual world, but there's always a chance something bad could happen to them. That's just life. In the event that your child does ever face a sexual crisis, you need to be prepared to take action. This chapter is about sexual emergencies: what to do if your child contracts an STD, gets pregnant (or gets his girlfriend pregnant), is in an abusive relationship, or gets sexually assaulted. Read through this now just to be prepared, but also keep in mind that you can use this section as a reference if one of these issues ever comes up.

Navigating Any Emergency

Although there are specific steps you should take for each of the individual emergencies listed in this chapter, there are also some general rules you can follow for the best way to react in any "sexual emergency" situation. Really, you can use these as guidelines for how to react any time your child tells you something that's hard for you to hear. Follow these steps to be able to respond to any emergency in a supportive, loving, and understanding way.

Step 1
Expect the Unexpected

Consider the statistics cited in previous chapters: half of all people contract an STD before they turn twenty-five, one in three teens gets pregnant before she turns twenty, one in six women are victims of a completed or attempted rape, and one in five teens has been physically struck by their partner. More than likely, your teen will experience some type of sexual emergency. In order to stay out of panic mode and be able to react calmly, expect that one day your teen is going to tell you some tough news. But also expect he or she may be in a crisis situation and *not* come to you. Part of expecting the unexpected is being on the lookout for signs that something unusual or upsetting is going on in your child's life.

Step 2
It's Not about You

Shit happens. Shit happens in every type of family to every type of kid. It doesn't mean you screwed up as a parent. Maybe you're upset. Maybe you're angry. Maybe you're frustrated, worried about how this will make you look, how this will make your family look, or what *your* parents will think. But take a deep breath before you react, and remember, this isn't about you. Your child is having an acute problem and needs your support and attention. The feelings you're having are important, but they aren't the main issue. You're doing a serious disservice to your teen if you let your emotions get in the way of helping your child through a rough situation. So push your own feelings aside to deal with later, bite your tongue if you have to, and focus a caring gaze onto your teen.

Step 3
React Thoughtfully

When your child is facing some sort of crisis, it's a time when he or she needs your love and support the most. "It is a critical moment in the relationship," cautions crisis counselor Louise Miller Lavin. "Be careful what words you choose because you can't erase them later. Your child will remember how you reacted in the heat of the moment. Keep in mind your ultimate goal through all of this is to move forward." More bluntly, this is not the time to reject, judge, criticize, or lecture your child. What's done is done, and if you react in anger, not only might your teen hold that against you, but he or she is not likely to seek your support again. The best way you can react is with love and understanding. Explicitly say, "I love you, and I will be here to help you in every way I can." Then reassure your child that you'll work together to get through this, and that it will be okay.

Step 4
Take Action

When your child is in an emergency situation, your role isn't necessarily to solve everything yourself, it's to get your child in touch with trained professionals who are best equipped to help: therapists, counselors, doctors, support groups or anyone else who might be able to offer assistance. With any sexual emergency, some choices are going to have to be made. But there's no rush to make them right away. In the heat of the moment, tell your child not to worry about making any decisions but to just stay open; discuss all of the options with a professional, and then make an educated choice later. Keep in mind that while you can help your child think about possible options, it's never your job to make the decision for him or her. You are there for guidance, not to make the final call.

Step 5
Beware of the Aftermath

Rarely does a crisis come without baggage. Although the situation itself may be over, chances are there will be emotions that linger. Make sure that you keep a close eye on your child. Continue to ask how it's going or if he or she wants to talk about what happened. As time goes on, be on the lookout for signs that things are not okay or that he or she is depressed. Does your teen seem quieter than usual or more withdrawn? Is he or she pulling away from friends? Are your child's grades slipping or are favorite activities being neglected? As well as enlisting the help of a therapist for guidance during a crisis, it may be helpful to have your child continue seeing someone after the crisis is over to help him or her through the recovery process.

What to Do If Your Child Gets an STD

The most important thing to remember about STDs is that they are very common. So while getting diagnosed with one will certainly feel like a crisis at the time, your child will learn how to live with the STD (or if they've contracted a curable one, they'll simply get it treated).

The Signs

From a parent's perspective, figuring out if your child has an STD is fairly straightforward. If your child comes to you concerned about possibly having one (whether it's because he or she had unprotected sex, is experiencing abnormal symptoms, or finds out a past partner has an STD), make a doctor's appointment for a full STD screening. You also have the choice of bringing your child to an STD clinic, or a Planned Parenthood office. Once you've gotten the results you'll know if he or she has an STD, or if an STD is a possibility (for limitations on STD testing please see Chapter 5).

What to Do at the Time

If your child just got diagnosed with an STD, he or she is likely to be terrified. The term "sexually transmitted disease" just sounds awful. The good news is, many STDs are completely curable (gonorrhea, chlamydia, crabs, and syphilis), so your first order of business should be to find out if the STD your child has can be cured. If it can be, reassure him or her that it will go away with treatment, and although it's scary, it's good that the infection was caught early. If your child is diagnosed with an STD that cannot be cured (HPV or herpes), reassure him or her that the STD can be managed.

Next, take the time to learn about the disease your child has been diagnosed with. "Knowing your child has something is just the beginning," says Linda Brown, MPH, an STD specialist for the South Carolina State Health Department. "It is important to understand what that disease is, what it will do to your child's body, what it will do to his or her fertility, and the best way to avoid passing it on to someone else." Unfortunately, many STD diagnoses go like this: "You have HPV. Your co-pay is fifteen dollars." Doctors don't always take the time to explain exactly what the disease is and what it means for someone's romantic future. Use the Internet to go to a credible website about the STD your child has (*www.ashastd.org* or *www.cdc.gov/std* are two good ones). There you can learn about treatment options, the disease implications, and what can be done to reduce the chances of transmission. You may also want to make a second doctor's appointment where your teen can go in with a list of questions and concerns he or she has about the STD.

Often the scariest thing about STDs for teens is the stigma attached to them. They may worry that everyone will think they're gross, or dirty, or that they'll suddenly become unlovable (be sure to tell your child none of this is true). Also make it clear that STDs are something that *many* people deal with in their lifetime. According to some experts I've spoken with, they believe almost everyone who is sexually active has been exposed to HPV. Telling your child that many—if not most—people get an STD at some point in their lifetime will help your child feel more normal, and less like a leper. You may even want to look up an exact statistic about how many people have the same STD, because it's likely a much higher number than your child assumes. (The STD Guide in the back of this book has some statistics listed.)

Stay calm, and if your child has an incurable STD, reassure him or her that it can be dealt with and it's possible to continue to lead a normal, happy, and healthy life. Although it may feel overwhelming right now, your child will get past this and move on.

Please note: *If your child is diagnosed with HIV, you may want to have him or her see a therapist who is trained to help people cope with their HIV-positive status.*

Moving Forward

The two most important things that people with an incurable STD need to understand are that having an STD may make them more vulnerable to contracting HIV (so they need to be extra careful about using condoms), and that having an STD means they are responsible for disclosing it to all of their future sex partners. You may want to have your child speak with a counselor or therapist about the best way to tell a future sexual partner that he or she has an STD. You can also help your teen think about what to say, although asking, "How are you going to tell your next special friend that you have sores on your wee wee," may be treading awfully close to the TMI line. So just be careful with the wording you use.

Something else that either you or a therapist may want to help your child think about is how the STD was contracted in the first place. And by "think about," I don't mean getting angry and berating him or her for having sex or for not using a condom. STDs can be contracted even when using a condom, so it may be that your teen did do everything possible to avoid STDs. But if he or she got an STD because a condom was not used, encourage your child to explore why that happened. Was it your child's choice not to use a condom? Or was your child giving in to pressure from his or her partner? And if that is the case, help your teen think about what it will it take to be stronger and more assertive next time around.

What to Do If Your Child Has an Unplanned Pregnancy

If your daughter becomes pregnant she will have three choices: have an abortion, carry the baby to term, or carry the baby to term and choose adoption. Although as a parent you will likely be involved in any decision she makes, it's important you understand that this is *her* decision. Your job isn't to make it for her, it is to support her afterward.

The Signs

The most telling sign that your daughter is pregnant is if she misses her period. But girls can also skip their period for a variety of other reasons: stress, change in diet, change in exercise patterns, weight loss, weight gain, and the list goes on. A girl who is pregnant may also experience morning sickness, sore breasts, dizziness, feeling the constant urge to pee, or having cramps without actually getting a period.

If your daughter comes to you worried that she is pregnant, have her take a pregnancy test (you can buy them at any drug store). The best tests are the ones that have two boxes. One of the boxes reports if the test was used correctly, and the other one reports if a girl is pregnant or not. Do make sure that no matter what type of test you are using, you read the instructions and your daughter follows them correctly.

What to Do at the Time

If you find out your daughter is pregnant, first and foremost don't freak out (at least on the outside). This isn't the time to yell or lecture or make your daughter feel shameful about what happened. Like any other bump in the road, immediately tell your daughter that you love her, that you will help her, and that you will support any decision she makes regarding the pregnancy. Also let her know she doesn't have to make that decision right away. She should take some time to speak with someone, reflect on her options, and decide what is best for her.

After comforting your daughter, go into action mode and find a pregnancy counselor who can speak with her about all of the alternatives. Planned Parenthood has pregnancy counselors on staff that are trained for this exact situation and can give girls unbiased information about all of their options. Beware of "crisis pregnancy centers," organizations set up for the sole purpose of discouraging girls from having abortions. A sign that a clinic is a crisis pregnancy center is if it's listed in the phone book under "abortion alternatives," or if no one will give you a clear answer about what services they offer or the nature of their counseling. Any legitimate counseling center will be up front about the fact that they provide nonjudgmental information and help girls consider all of their options.

The three options your daughter has are: to have an abortion, to carry the baby to term and choose adoption, to or carry the baby to term and care for it herself. If she is going to have an abortion, she must decide to do so within the first few months of becoming pregnant. If she decides to have one within the first nine weeks, she has the most options available for the type of abortion that she can have. If your daughter is going to have the baby (or there is any chance she might decide to), it's important that she gets prenatal care ASAP. Make an appointment with a doctor who can advise her on how to keep the baby healthy. If she drinks, smokes, or is taking any type of nonprescription drug, she must stop immediately.

If you have a son who has gotten a girl pregnant, in a way your role is trickier because ultimately he's not the one who is going to be making the decision. He's just going to have to deal with whatever decision is made. There is no clear-cut best way to help your son deal with an unplanned pregnancy because each situation is different. "Some boys may need to be reminded that they have a responsibility for the pregnancy too, while other boys who are more sensitive and emotionally involved may just have to be comforted," says crisis counselor Louise Miller Lavin. "It's hard to know what to tell your son to do because some families may want no contact from the father, whereas other families will expect him to reach out to help deal with the situation emotionally as well as financially." You may simply want to make sure your son has let the girl know his help is available if she wants it, and from there, just roll with the punches.

Moving Forward

You might think that a girl who has gotten pregnant once has "learned her lesson," but studies show that many people who have abortions have more than one—suggesting they are continuing to have trouble with contraception. No matter what your daughter decides to do about the unplanned pregnancy, you should make sure she has the resources to avoid another one in the future. Make an appointment with a doctor where she can explore her contraceptive options and choose one that is right for her. And if it's your son who was involved with an unplanned pregnancy, remind him that condoms not only protect against STDs, they also help prevent pregnancy. If your child (male or female) has any misconceptions about pregnancy ("you can't get pregnant on your period," or "'pulling out' is reliable contraception"), make sure he or she is set straight. Encourage your teen to learn from this mistake in order to avoid repeating it in the future.

Even as the unplanned pregnancy drifts further into the past, continue to be aware of any emotional support your child may still need. A young woman may still have to talk about the choice she made long after the incident has passed. And very likely, she will continue to want your reassurance that it was the right one. So remind her that she made the decision she did for a reason, and while it's easy to look back and question what she was thinking, when faced with the reality of a pregnancy, there was one answer that stood out as the best choice.

What to Do If Your Child Is in an Abusive Relationship

Although both guys and girls can be victims in an abusive relationship, the victims are overwhelmingly women, and the abusers are mostly men. For that reason, this section is written assuming the abuser is a "he," and the victim in the relationship is your daughter. But keep in mind as you read this, that when it comes to emotional and psychological abuse, the abuser can just as easily be a woman. Also keep in mind that abuse has no sexual orientation—gay teens (both male and female) can be in abusive relationships as well.

The Signs

Although you may not see exactly what goes on in your children's relationships, you should be aware of the way they are acting and what's going on in their lives in general. Those things can help serve as clues to the health of their intimate relationships. Some of the telltale signs that your daughter is in an abusive relationship are: she doesn't seem to be hanging out much with friends, she's stopped showing an interest in being around family, her grades are slipping, or she seems uninterested in hobbies that used to excite her. These are all indications that your daughter is becoming increasingly isolated, which is one of the things that an abusive partner tries to accomplish.

Another thing you can look for is a change in your child's overall demeanor and appearance. Does she always seem down or upset, or is she crying much more than usual? Has she made any comments or behaved in a way that might indicate she's afraid of her boyfriend? Has she suddenly started changing the way she dresses because her boyfriend wants her to dress a certain way? Physically, have you noticed any bruises, or does she seem to be "getting injured" often? If the way she's acting seems strange and out of character, take that as a warning that something is going on (be it in her relationship or otherwise).

Finally, there may be some things that you can tell about the relationship by observing her boyfriend's behavior. If she has a cell phone, chances are you pay the bill. I'm not necessarily advising you to snoop, but if you notice her boyfriend's number called excessively and repeatedly (because maybe she wasn't picking up), that could be a sign of controlling behavior. If you have seen him have violent outbursts and hit or throw things (even objects), take that as a warning he may have trouble controlling his emotions. And finally, observe the way he talks to her. Does he seem to disrespect her when they talk, put her down, act possessively, or constantly criticize her? Remember that abuse can be emotional and psychological as well as physical.

Emotional abuse is the main type of abuse to be aware of if you have a son. Notice if his girlfriend is trying to make him feel bad about himself, critiquing his every move, or seems overly possessive or demanding.

What to Do If You Suspect an Abusive Relationship

If you suspect that your daughter is in an abusive relationship, you should confront her about it—but in a nonconfrontational way. Keep in mind your ultimate goal: your daughter's safety and health. Your goal is *not* to get her to admit her boyfriend is abusive or concede that you were right all along and he's complete scum. Tell her you've noticed she seems upset and ask her if she wants to talk about it. You can also probe her by saying you know how involved she is with her boyfriend and asking if they are going through a rough spot or having any trouble getting along (this way, you don't come right out and accuse him). Remember that even if he is scum to you, this relationship is very real to her. She may be experiencing love for the first time, and she may feel very dedicated to and passionate about the relationship. Outwardly criticizing, accusing, or judging her boyfriend or their relationship is likely to just push her away.

Talk with your daughter "generally" about what a healthy relationship looks like. Tell her "love should not hurt" and explain what types of behaviors are unacceptable within a relationship (for a refresher go back to Chapter 3). This way, you're letting her know what may be happening to her is not okay, but you're not directly attacking her boyfriend. You can also give her the number for the national domestic abuse hotline: 1-800-799-SAFE (7233), and tell her if she ever has any questions about normal boyfriend behavior, she can ask a counselor on the hotline confidentially. She may feel more comfortable discussing her feelings with a stranger at first, and then involving you later.

If you think your daughter is in an abusive relationship, your first instinct may be to forbid her from seeing her boyfriend or to try to convince her to break up with him. But ultimately, the realization that a relationship is unhealthy and the decision to get out of it are conclusions she's going to have to come to herself.

If your daughter comes right out and tells you she is being abused, then your job is a little easier, since you don't have to worry about coming across as accusatory. Reaffirm that the way her boyfriend is treating her isn't right, and reassure her that there are many other guys out there who will treat her well. Tell her you "*strongly* advise" that she get out of the relationship and that you will be there to help her in every way possible when she does. But make clear that you will love and support her no matter what. The last thing you want is for your daughter to feel even more isolated by thinking you will be angry with her if she doesn't get out of the relationship quickly enough.

What to Do to Get Her to Leave

Even if you know your daughter is in an abusive relationship, you can't tell her she *has* to break up with her boyfriend because at the end of the day, that's just not something you can enforce. Your best move is to put all the pieces in place for her to make the easiest exit possible and then let her decide to make that exit when she's ready. You should work to rebuild the self-confidence that her boyfriend has likely torn down. Tell her how amazing, smart, beautiful, and loveable she is. Tell her how she's not that experienced now, but as she gets older she'll see how many great guys will want to date her. (If she's been getting emotionally abused, her boyfriend has likely tried to convince her that no one else would love her the way he does, or even that no one else would ever show interest in her.) As well as building up her self-confidence, you can encourage her to reconnect with friends or get more involved in things she used to enjoy. This way, she will remember she has a life outside of her boyfriend.

Jane Key, the sexual violence services coordinator for the South Carolina Department of Health says parents should "be there for their child, but not be judgmental. The goal is to open the door of communication, keep that door open, and keep talking. Remind your daughter that she is somebody, and she's somebody without her boyfriend." She also recommends that you enlist outside assistance to help your daughter deal with the situation. She may want to see a counselor or therapist, and when your daughter does leave her boyfriend, you may need to speak with her teachers or her guidance counselor to get her schedule changed if she's in any of the same classes as her abusive ex.

If your daughter has made the decision to leave, be very cautious of her safety, especially if her relationship is physically abusive. Know that when she breaks up with her boyfriend he could fly off the handle. She needs to make sure that she does it in a safe place and remains protected for the next few days until he calms down. For more tips and advice you may want to speak with someone at a local battered women's shelter or call the national domestic abuse hotline yourself. Again, that number is 1-800-799-7233.

Moving Forward

Although anyone can get into an abusive relationship, it's possible your daughter has confidence issues that kept her in the relationship, or even low self-confidence as a result of it. Those feelings may be something she wants to work through with the help of a therapist. Either you or a therapist should help her process what happened and figure out if there were any warning signs she ignored. Talk to your daughter about ways she can recognize a potentially abusive relationship from the beginning, and about the need to get out of it immediately.

You should also continue to build up her self-esteem (see Chapter 1 for details) and encourage her to expand her support network. Suggest that she reestablish friendships with people she may have distanced herself from while she was with her boyfriend. Do what you can to get her reinvolved in her favorite hobbies or pastimes. And remind her that she can always come to you with any problem, and that you'll always be there to help.

What to Do If Your Child Gets Sexually Assaulted

Similar to the previous section, although men can be sexually assaulted, more often than not, the victims of sexual assault are women and the assailants are men. For the purposes of this section, I'm assuming a young woman was assaulted, and a young man is the perpetrator.

The Signs

There may not be any explicit signs that your child has been sexually assaulted other than her coming right out and telling you. If she suddenly shows signs of depression or anxiety, starts doing drugs, or starts behaving abnormally in any other way, it's a sign that *something* serious is going on in her life. That something may or may not be a sexual assault, but regardless of the culprit, you should try to figure out what is going on, and what you can do to make it better.

What to Do at the Time

*Please note that all of the steps listed are to meet the immediate concerns of a girl's health and to **possibly** build a case against her attacker in the future. Whether or not she wants to formally press charges is a decision she can make later. Seeking medical attention in no way **requires** her to do so.*

If your daughter has just been raped, what you do immediately is important. Although her first instinct may be to shower, have her stay in the same clothes she is wearing. Should she decide that she wants to press charges, there may be incriminating evidence on her clothes and on her body. If she has already taken off her clothes, put them in a clean *paper* bag. If your daughter feels up to it, have her write down any of the details she remembers from the attack. Again, those details can help her *if* she decides to press charges.

Next, you have the option of calling the national sexual assault hotline (1-800-656-HOPE). The hotline is answered twenty-four hours a day by counselors who can give you immediate instructions on what to do. The counselor can also see if there is a rape crisis center in your area.

Whether or not you call the hotline, your next step is to make sure your daughter gets prompt medical attention. The best bet is to take her to the ER at any hospital. In the ER, ask if there is a SANE nurse on staff (Sexual Assault Nurse Examiner). SANE nurses are specially trained to care for rape victims and help comfort them during a rape kit exam. During this exam, evidence is taken from a girl's body and clothing and is then held confidentially. If *and only if* she decides she wants to press charges against her attacker, the evidence collected during the exam can be used. Your daughter does not have to get a rape kit exam, but if she does, there is a much higher chance that her assailant will get convicted if she decides to press charges.

Even if your daughter doesn't want the exam, or there isn't a SANE nurse available, she should still see a health care provider. During the assault she may have been put at risk for an unplanned pregnancy, STDs, or even HIV. Your daughter may need to take emergency contraception, and if she's worried she was exposed to HIV, there is a medication she can take within the first thirty-six hours to help reduce her risk of contracting the virus. She also needs to be examined to see if she was injured in any way during the assault.

In the initial hours after the attack, tell your daughter not to worry about whether or not she wants to press charges against her attacker. That is something she can deal with later. Because the assault is likely swirling around her head, keep letting her know that she is safe now and that you will help her get through this. Also let her know that what happened was in no way her fault.

Don't push your daughter to press charges. Depending on the situation, she may not feel it's worth it. Often rape victims are completely dragged through the mud for accusing someone (especially if it's someone they know) of rape. The sad reality is, even if there is lots of evidence to back her up, her peers may still torture her for the accusation. Remember, the most important thing is that she be able to recover as quickly as possible, not that "that SOB hears from my lawyer."

Moving Forward

A friend of mine was raped, and she said that although people were very supportive the first week, as time went on everyone seemed to forget about it. After a month they acted like she should "just be over it already." But she wasn't over it, and while her friends may have put it out of their minds, she continued to deal with the assault for years afterward.

It takes many women a long time to recover from a sexual assault. Some victims develop depression, posttraumatic stress disorder, drug addictions, anxiety disorders, and eating disorders. Especially right after the assault, your daughter may experience severe flashbacks, anxiety, and depression. And she may have to be in counseling for some time to help her work through those issues. Don't expect your daughter to be "back to normal" after a month or two, but know that she will show improvement over time. Even years later, you need to stay tuned in to her behavior and be alert for signs of anxiety, depression, or drug addiction. Keep supporting her, keep talking to her, and keep encouraging her. She will get better.

Time does heal, but it can do so slowly. With any sort of crisis your child is facing, just be loving and supportive—when in doubt about how to act, you can never go wrong with that.

Chapter Eleven
NO MATTER WHAT, YOU CAN DO IT

Parents may not be the primary sex educators of their children, but they can still give their children clear positive messages about their bodies and teach them how to honor and relate to people. Even if parents aren't content specialists, they can still be moral educators.

—Robert Blum, MD, PhD, MPH, Johns Hopkins University

Maybe you'll never be the parent that corners your kid with a banana and a box of condoms. And that's okay. Many of the things that will help a child's sexual health the most have more to do with values than the nuts and bolts of intercourse. No matter how squeamish you may be about sex, you can talk with your kids about what a healthy relationship looks like and teach them they deserve a partner who treats them well and looks out for their needs. Any parent can instill a sense of respect for other people and other people's boundaries. And no matter how prudish you may be, you can help your kids filter through the damaging messages they see in the media.

There's a lot of information in this book, and it may be a bit overwhelming. Don't worry, I'm not expecting that you'll memorize all of it and recite every word back to your teens. Your kids aren't doomed if you don't discuss every topic in here. But at least you have that option.

Teens need to know how to counter complaints about condoms. They need to know that most STDs aren't obvious, that oral sex is sex, and that there are many safe and effective forms of contraception available. But many kids never get this information. Not in school, not from their doctors, and certainly not from their friends. Someone needs to talk with them about these things. Now, that person can be you. Or maybe you want to dole that responsibility out to their older sibling, an aunt or uncle, a cousin, a close family friend, or a trusted physician.

But no matter who else talks to your kids about sex or how few sexual topics you are willing to broach yourself, you still have a lot of responsibilities. Relax, because it won't be embarrassing to fulfill them. Your primary job is to build a close relationship with your teens, shape their values, and raise their self-esteem. These are the basic things every parent *can* and should do to make sure their teens approach sex and relationships in a healthy way.

Stay Connected

Remain close with your kids as they become teenagers. Your kids enjoy spending time with you, they respect your opinion, and they value your advice (even though they may not always act like it). A friend of mine says that throughout some of the backstabbing friends she had in high school, she always knew the one person who would always have her best interest in mind was her mother. As a parent, you matter much more to your kids than their friends.

Stay involved in your children's life. Not in a prying way, but because you care about what's going on. Know who they are hanging out with, notice what their friends are like, and which friends aren't in their life anymore. If they start dating, get them to talk about their relationship and about their partner. Show interest in meeting their significant other because you want to meet the person they care so much about (not because you question their judgment). And keep reinforcing the qualities that make a good mate, and a healthy relationship.

The better connected you are with your kids, the better you'll be able to recognize when something in their life is going wrong. You'll know when they're not acting like themselves, or when they're showing signs of distress. And the closer you are to your children, the better you'll be able to make a difference when they are in bad situations.

Be Aware of Open Doors

Actively pay attention to what your children are reading, watching, and listening to, and listen to it with them. If there's something sexual in the content, don't turn it off or ignore it, take that as an opportunity to start a conversation. If there is a news story about a serial rapist, talk with your kids about the fact that date rape is actually much more common. If you can't pry the fashion magazines out of your daughter's hands, point to some of the super-skinny models and remind her that being that thin isn't healthy.

Most importantly, pay attention when your kids bring up a conversation or drop hints that they want to talk about something—and strike while the iron is hot. If your daughter is making comments that suggest she is thinking about sexual orientation, start a conversation then and there. Don't say you'll talk about it later, because that door is open now, and it may not open again anytime soon. When talking with your children about sexual issues, you're going to have to play on their court, when they're ready.

Be a Good Listener

I had an art teacher in middle school who would always say, "Draw what you see, not what you know." Listen to your kids the same way. What are they actually saying to you? (Not what do you suspect they mean by it.) If you're not sure what exactly they're saying, ask them to clarify. Notice what concerns they are expressing and address them, even if they seem irrelevant or unimportant to you. If you can't, think about who could.

Part of being a good listener is creating an environment where your kids feel comfortable talking. This means not being judgmental when they tell you something. If your eighth-grade son tells you his friend was talking about blowjobs and you yell back at him, "That's totally inappropriate! That kid is never coming over here again!" you're not creating a say-anything safe zone. Keep an open mind, and watch how you respond when your teen tells you something. Maybe that means counting to three in your head, taking a deep breath, and digging your nails into your palms before you say anything (if that is what it takes to respond calmly). If you need to go ape-shit about something your kid said, do it later after he or she has left the room. Your ultimate goal is to be such a good listener your child knows you can be consulted about anything.

Don't Be a Friend, but Be a Friendly Parent

If your kids are running around yelling "rim job" and drawing penises on foggy glass, you don't have to be going around doing it with them. Your job isn't to be "cool parent," letting anything go and chiming in when they talk about sex in a casual or destructive way. By all means do everything you can to relate to your kids, talk in a language they understand, and give them realistic advice. But don't cross the line and talk to them the same way you would talk to a friend—that's the type of approach that leads to TMI moments. Although you don't want to be overly critical, you can still talk to your children as a parent and offer them boundaries.

Make an effort to be a warm and friendly resource for your kids. Tell them you're happy to answer any question they may have about sex and relationships. Make sure they know that when they're ready to become sexually active, you will be there to help them with contraception or to take them to a doctor. Reassure them that no matter what kind of situation they are in, they can always come to you for guidance, and you will always be there to help.

You don't have to be Dr. Ruth to be able to help your teens with sex—you just have to be a good parent. Support your kids and make them feel good about themselves. Teach them to value and respect their bodies and to always demand that others do the same. And of course, you can't forget to tell them the most important thing of all—that you'll always love them very much. It is with that foundation that your kids will make the most fulfilling sexual choices, pursue healthy romantic relationships, and one day—when they've *planned* it—have a happy family of their own.

APPENDIX A: SEXUALLY TRANSMITTED DISEASES AND VAGINAL INFECTIONS GUIDE

The information in this guide isn't meant to serve as a substitute for taking your child to a doctor if he or she is experiencing unusual genital symptoms or is for whatever reason worried about having an STD. Instead, I've included these descriptions so that you can use this book as an initial reference should a health question arise. The STDs outlined here are the most common/threatening STDs that your child may be exposed to after becoming sexually active. I have not included a description of Hepatitis B, since the vast majority of kids receive the extremely effective vaccine. If you don't think yours has, or you are at all unsure, check in with their doctor, and have them get the vaccination ASAP.

After this STD Guide is a Vaginal Infections Guide, since it's very likely that if your daughter is complaining about an odd vaginal symptom, it could be coming from an infection, rather than an STD. But of course, only a visit to the doctor's office will be able to determine that for sure. Please note that all of the STDs and vaginal infections are listed alphabetically.

STDs

CHLAMYDIA

What it is: A bacterial sexually transmitted disease that often has no symptoms but can permanently damage a woman's reproductive system if left untreated.

How common it is: Chlamydia is the most commonly reported bacterial STD—about one million cases a year. But because people with chlamydia often have no symptoms, the actual number of cases each year is likely much higher (CDC Chlamydia Fact Sheet 2009). The southeastern United States has a much higher rate of chlamydia than the rest of the country, so if you live in the southeast, chlamydia should be of particular concern. Also, girls under twenty are particularly vulnerable to these bacteria.

Of note: Although chlamydia can be easily treated with antibiotics, if left untreated in women, 40 percent of the time it will lead to pelvic inflammatory disease (CDC 2009). Pelvic inflammatory disease can permanently damage a woman's reproductive system leading to chronic pelvic pain, complications with pregnancy, and infertility. Even once the infection is treated, any damage it has caused cannot be reversed.

How it's contracted: Chlamydia can be spread through vaginal or anal intercourse and very rarely oral sex. Using a condom greatly reduces one's chance of contracting chlamydia, since the disease is transmitted through infected sexual fluids.

Signs and symptoms: Most people who experience symptoms do so within one to three weeks of becoming infected. Only about half of men who are infected with chlamydia experience any symptoms, which can include a burning sensation when they pee, itching around the opening of the penis, and a discharge dripping out of the penis. Only about a quarter of women experience symptoms from chlamydia, and the rest notice nothing. Women who do experience symptoms may notice burning when they pee or a change in the smell or consistency of their vaginal discharge. More advanced infections that have spread to other organs may cause lower abdominal pain, back pain, pain during intercourse, bleeding between periods, and possibly even fever and nausea.

Getting tested: For men and women there are both swab tests and urine tests that can check for chlamydia.

Treatment: Chlamydia can be treated with a simple course of antibiotics. In order to avoid reinfection, both sex partners should be treated and refrain from any sexual activity until they are finished taking all of their pills and have both tested negative for the bacteria. (The last thing they want to do is keep reinfecting each other.)

CRABS/PUBIC LICE

What it is: Crabs, aka pubic lice, are very similar to head lice, except that they live in the coarse hair on someone's body (pubic hair, chest hair, armpit hair, and even eyebrows and eye lashes).

How common it is: Pubic lice is a fairly common STD; there are about 3 million cases reported every year (CDC 2009).

Of note: Although having crabs may be uncomfortable, they won't cause any serious damage—aside from the headache of treating them.

How it's contracted: Like head lice, pubic lice is *very* contagious. One can contract it through any sort of intimate contact, or even sharing clothing (generally a bathing suit or underwear), sharing towels, or sleeping in an infected person's bed. Using a condom is always a good idea, but condoms don't do anything to prevent the spread of pubic lice.

Signs and symptoms: It usually takes about five days for someone to begin experiencing symptoms from pubic lice. But unlike the majority of STDs, almost everybody infected does experience noticeable symptoms. Someone with crabs will likely notice an itchy pubic region, and upon close inspection may even see the actual lice or their eggs. Pubic lice look like small light-gray or rust-colored dots, and the eggs are more of an off-white color.

Getting tested: Since pubic lice are visible, many people just diagnose themselves. But one can also go to a doctor, health department, or a Planned Parenthood clinic if he or she wants a professional opinion.

Treatment: Just like head lice, getting rid of pubic lice is a bit of a hassle. In order to get rid of all the possible lice and their eggs, everything must be washed in extremely hot water, and anything that can't be washed must be bagged up for two weeks. As far as treating the lice on one's body, all infected regions should be washed with a special lice-killing shampoo. That shampoo can be bought at most pharmacies as an over-the-counter medication. Like any curable STD, all partners should be treated before any sexual activity is resumed.

GONORRHEA

What it is: Gonorrhea is a bacterial sexually transmitted disease that can also affect the anus and throat and damage both males' and females' reproductive organs if left untreated.

How common it is: Gonorrhea is the second-most-common bacterial STD—right behind chlamydia—an estimated 700,000 people are infected with gonorrhea every year (CDC 2009).

Of note: People who have gonorrhea often have chlamydia as well, so anyone who tests positive for gonorrhea should also be tested for chlamydia. If left untreated, a gonorrheal infection can cause pelvic inflammatory disease in women (which can result in chronic pelvic pain, infertility, and ectopic pregnancies) as well as epididymitis in men—which can be both painful and cause infertility. An untreated infection can also spread to the blood or joints, which can be life threatening.

How it's contracted: Gonorrhea can be spread through vaginal and anal intercourse as well as oral sex. Using a condom greatly reduces one's risk of contracting this infection.

Signs and symptoms: Many guys who contract gonorrhea develop symptoms within a few days, although for some it takes as long as a month, and others don't have any symptoms at all. Those who do have symptoms may experience burning when they pee, have sore or swollen testicles, or have a whitish, yellowish, or greenish discharge dripping from the penis (hence the name, "the drip"). The majority of women who contract gonorrhea don't have any symptoms at all, and those who do often have ones that are very minor. Those symptoms might include burning when peeing, pain when having sex, bleeding in between periods, or a sore or swollen vagina. People infected with gonorrhea in their anus may experience pain or itching when they are going to the bathroom, and those with gonorrhea of the throat may have a sore throat. In general, those with gonorrhea of the throat or anus don't notice anything.

Getting tested: A guy or girl can easily be tested for gonorrhea by having either a penile or cervical swab. And if someone is having symptoms in their mouth or anus they can have an oral or anal swab done as well. There is also a urine test that can screen for genital infections.

Treatment: Just like chlamydia, gonorrhea can be treated with antibiotics. Also like chlamydia, any damage that has been caused by an untreated infection will not go away with antibiotics. In order to avoid reinfection, it's important that all sex partners have finished treatment and have both tested negative for gonorrhea before any sexual activity is resumed.

HERPES

What it is: Herpes is a virus that causes sores either around the mouth or around the genitals. Herpes type 1 mainly causes sores around the mouth (although it *can* cause sores on the genitals), and herpes type 2 causes sores around the genitals.

How common it is: In the United States, it's estimated that one out of five people over age twelve have genital herpes. Genital herpes is also more common in women; about one out of four women (and only about one out of eight men) have genital herpes (CDC 2009).

Of note: Sometimes, a person with genital herpes can give his or her partner mouth sores from oral sex. Similarly, a person with oral herpes can give a partner genital sores from oral sex. Because of this crossover, someone with an active herpes sore on his or her mouth should not be performing oral sex, and someone with an active herpes sore on his or her genitals should not be receiving oral sex. Even if there isn't an active sore, since infected skin (with no visible symptoms) can still carry the virus, when having oral sex, it is safest to always use a condom or an oral dam.

How it's contracted: Genital herpes can be spread through vaginal or anal intercourse (as well as oral sex—explained above). Using a condom will greatly reduce the risk of spreading or contracting herpes. As with HPV, however, since a condom does not cover the entire area that might have a herpes sore, one can still get herpes when having protected sex. Also similar to HPV, since herpes is spread through skin-to-skin contact, it can be passed on simply by two people rubbing against each other naked (when no other sex act has taken place).

The herpes virus is most contagious when there is an active sore. However, most people contract herpes from a partner who does not know he or she is infected and has no visible signs of the virus.

Signs and symptoms: Many people with genital herpes may have such mild symptoms that they never know they have it, or don't find out until years later. Those who do get herpes sores may get them anywhere on or around their genitals, anus, butt, or even on their thighs. The first outbreak of herpes is usually the most severe. During the first outbreak (likely to occur within two weeks of when someone contracted the virus), one or more painful blisters appear around the genital area, and the infected person may run a fever or experience other flu-like symptoms. But not all herpes blisters are obvious. Many people who have herpes mistake their blisters for something else, like a rash, cuts, bumps, razor burn, hemorrhoids, or, for girls, a yeast infection.

Getting tested: Usually, if someone wants to get tested for herpes, he or she visits the doctor when a blister is present. The doctor can then either visually diagnose the sore, or swab it and test the sample for the herpes virus. There is also a blood test for herpes, but this test is pretty rarely offered because it's pretty rarely requested. It's not requested because someone who has never had any herpes symptoms and tests positive doesn't know what to do with the results. Although the virus is somewhere in their body, they've never seen evidence of it, so what do they say to their future partners?

Treatment: Although herpes sores can be treated, the virus that causes them remains in the body forever, and outbreaks may continue for the rest of a person's life. The first year that someone is infected is generally the worst, and one can expect about four or five outbreaks. After the initial year, herpes outbreaks are likely to become less frequent.

As for the herpes sores themselves, they can be treated with an oral medication that will shorten the duration of the outbreak and hopefully make it less painful. Oral medications can also be taken daily to decrease the frequency and severity of the outbreaks (which has the added benefit of making the virus less contagious). And if someone is having a particularly painful outbreak, a doctor can prescribe a cream to help lessen the pain.

HIV/AIDS

What it is: HIV, human immunodeficiency virus, is a virus that attacks a person's T cells (necessary for a healthy immune system) and eventually progresses into acquired immunodeficiency syndrome (AIDS). A person who is HIV positive has AIDS once their T cell count falls below 200, or when they develop an AIDS-related illness. People who are infected with HIV can seem completely healthy for years until they develop AIDS, at which point they become very sick (since their immune system is severely compromised).

How common it is: According to the CDC (Centers for Disease Control and Prevention), someone in the United States is infected with HIV every nine and a half minutes, and more infections occur in young people ages thirteen to twenty-nine than any other age group (2008). The CDC now estimates that only about half of HIV positive young people are actually aware they are infected (2009). HIV infection rates continue to remain high in the gay and bisexual male population, as well as in African American men and women (CDC 2008).

Of note: It is possible to have sex with someone who is HIV positive and not contract the virus. For this reason, just because someone has engaged in unprotected sex once, it does not mean that what's done is done and they may as well do it again. Each act of unprotected sex puts someone at a new risk for HIV and all STDs.

How it's contracted: Aside from sharing needles, HIV is spread through unprotected vaginal and anal sex. Although it's possible to contract HIV through unprotected oral sex, that is fairly rare. You cannot get HIV by hugging, kissing, sharing food with, sitting next to, or otherwise interacting with someone who is infected. Using a condom greatly reduces one's chances of contracting HIV.

Signs and symptoms: When someone first contracts the HIV virus, he or she may develop flu-like symptoms within a few days or weeks. After that, it could be over a decade before someone with HIV notices anything abnormal. Someone whose HIV infection has progressed may eventually experience dramatic weight loss, fatigue, swollen lymph nodes, a dry cough, diarrhea, night sweats, or pneumonia. Women may also experience frequent vaginal infections, pelvic inflammatory disease, and abnormal pap smears.

Getting tested: There are several different ways to test for HIV. Some tests use mouth swabs, and others use blood. There are rapid tests available that give results in twenty minutes, and others can take a few days or even two weeks. Because the majority of tests screen for the body's reaction to the HIV virus, people must wait a while after possible exposure in order to get an accurate result. Doctors recommend that people wait at least two months before getting tested. And to get the most accurate reading, a person should get tested again after six months.

Treatment: The HIV virus cannot be cured, although there are many drugs available that can help those infected live longer and stay healthier. In fact, the majority of HIV positive people who take these medications may never develop AIDS. These treatments, however, are by no means a magic bullet, must be taken every day for the rest of one's life, and often have side effects. But new research continues to be done, and hopefully within our lifetimes we will see new ways to prevent, manage, and possibly cure the virus.

HPV

What it is: HPV (human papillomavirus) is the virus that causes cervical cancer and genital warts. There are over thirty strains of the virus that affect the genital area, and each strain may cause either warts or cervical cancer, but not both. Anyone who has both symptoms is infected with two different strains of the virus. Warts do not turn into cervical cancer, and cervical cancer doesn't turn into warts. One of the biggest risks of HPV is that an infected person may or may not show symptoms, but can still pass it on.

How common it is: Some statistics suggest that at least 50 percent of sexually active men and women will contract HPV at some point in their lifetime (CDC 2009). Other sources believe that number is closer to 80 percent since many people who have HPV may never know they have it.

Of note: The HPV vaccine, Gardasil (currently recommended for girls ages nine to twelve or any female under the age of twenty-six who has not been vaccinated, and an option for boys as well), protects people from four strains of the HPV virus. Those four strains are responsible for 70 percent of cervical cancer cases, and 90 percent of genital warts cases. Even if a girl receives the vaccine, she should still get pap-smears and HPV DNA tests since the vaccine doesn't protect against all strains of HPV. Giving your son the HPV vaccine will help protect him against genital warts and also help ensure he won't be a carrier for the types of HPV that cause cancer.

How it's contracted: HPV can be spread through vaginal, anal, and even oral sex. Because warts can be present anywhere in the "boxer shorts" area, the strains of HPV that cause warts can be spread simply by two people rubbing their pelvic regions against each other naked. Using a condom greatly reduces the risk of spreading or contracting HPV. But since a condom doesn't cover the entire boxer shorts area, the strains of HPV that can cause genital warts can still be passed on even if a condom is used. It's important to note that the HPV virus is more contagious at times when the person carrying it has warts versus times when he or she does not.

Signs and symptoms: One of the biggest problems with HPV is that it can be so hard to detect. Young men who are carrying a strain of HPV that may cause cancer have no signs or symptoms. Young women who are carrying a cancer-causing strain also have no symptoms—although they can at least get tested by getting a pap smear and/or an HPV DNA test. *Some* people who are infected with a strain of HPV that causes genital warts develop warts anywhere in or around their genitals, anus, or upper-thigh area. Others don't develop warts at all (although they can still pass on the virus). If warts do develop, they will likely do so a few weeks to a few months after someone is infected. Warts are small grayish, whitish, or flesh-colored painless bumps that can appear in groups or singly. If left untreated, the warts may disappear on their own, stay the same, or get bigger or multiply. Because the warts are painless and oftentimes subtle, many people either don't notice them or mistake them for an ingrown hair or random skin bump and never see a doctor about it.

Getting tested: There is no test for men that can detect the strains of HPV that can cause cancer. Sexually active young women can get pap-smears and HPV DNA tests to see if they have a strain of HPV that causes cervical cancer. Genital warts themselves can be visually diagnosed by a doctor. Some doctors use an acidic solution on the genital area that helps very small or flat warts become more visible.

Treatment: A girl whose pap smear comes back abnormal doesn't have cervical cancer, she has the beginning of a condition that if left untreated may become cancer. If a girl has an abnormal pap smear, she may either get more frequent pap smears (to monitor the situation), or the abnormal cells on the cervix may be cut off or frozen. A guy or girl who has genital warts can have the warts burned or frozen off, apply a cream to make them go away, or let them go away on their own. But as long as the HPV virus remains in the body, new warts may appear sporadically, even after the old ones have gone away.

Although the symptoms of the HPV virus can be treated, the virus itself cannot be cured, and stays in the body for some time. In many cases, it goes away on its own after a year or two (after the body's immune system has fought it off). But since it is not always possible to determine when the virus has left, there is no way for a guy to say for sure he no longer has HPV, and there's no way for a girl to say for sure she no longer has a strain of HPV that cause warts. (By having an HPV DNA test, a girl can determine when she no longer has a strain of HPV that causes cervical cancer.)

SYPHILIS

What it is: Syphilis is a fairly uncommon curable bacterial STD that can be life threatening if left untreated.

How common it is: Until recently, syphilis was extremely rare. But lately, rates have been rising in certain populations. Gay and bisexual men, African Americans, and people in the southeastern United States are at the highest risk for contracting this STD.

How it's contracted: Syphilis is contracted mainly through unprotected vaginal or anal intercourse. It can also be contracted through unprotected oral sex, but that is fairly uncommon. Syphilis is generally spread through direct contact with a syphilis sore (usually on the vagina, penis, or anus, and possibly around the mouth). The sore (or chancre, pronounced "shanker") is a symptom of the first stage of syphilis, and when it is present, the disease is the most contagious. Like many STDs, using a condom greatly reduces one's risk of contracting it.

Signs and symptoms: There are three stages of syphilis, and each one is marked by different signs and symptoms. Someone is contagious, however, only in the first and second stages. The first stage usually occurs within a few weeks of when someone was exposed to the virus, but it can take as long as a few months. This phase is marked by the appearance of a chancre, which is a round, painless sore (occasionally a group of sores) that's usually somewhere around the genital area. The sore will go away on its own after a few weeks. The second stage of syphilis may begin when the original sore is healing or even months later. It consists of a rough, reddish-brown rash that's often on the palms of the hands or soles of the feet, and possibly other areas of the body. Syphilis is often called "the great imitator," because this rash is commonly mistaken for eczema, chicken pox, or other skin problems. Sometimes, the rash is accompanied by a fever and other flu-like symptoms. Like the first stage, the second stage will disappear on its own.

If syphilis is allowed to progress to the third stage, it can cause serious damage to one's body. The signs and symptoms of the late stage of syphilis can occur as late as ten to twenty years after infection and affect the heart, brain, liver, bones, blood vessels, and eyes. The symptoms may include severe lack of coordination, numbness, blindness, being unable to move, dementia, and possibly death. Although syphilis can be treated at any point it is detected, any damage it has already caused to internal organs cannot be undone.

Getting tested: There are many different widely available blood tests that can detect syphilis.

Treatment: Once diagnosed, the treatment for syphilis is easy: a course of penicillin.

VAGINAL INFECTIONS

Vaginal infections are a common problem that women deal with their entire lives. It's not unusual for a girl to freak out that she has an STD when she in fact has a vaginal infection. On that same note, it's also not uncommon for a girl to mistake an STD for a vaginal infection, since many of the signs and symptoms are the same. For that reason, it's good to be aware of the most common vaginal infections. But a good rule of thumb, no matter what a girl's symptoms may be, if your daughter comes to you complaining about discomfort in her vagina, it's best to take her to a doctor so that the problem can be accurately diagnosed.

YEAST INFECTIONS

What it is: If you're a woman, chances are you've had a yeast infection. A yeast infection is just an overgrowth of yeast (a type of fungus) that is naturally in the vagina.

What causes it: Although there is no specific cause of yeast infections, taking antibiotics, hormone fluctuations, wearing tight clothing that doesn't breathe (like spandex), or wearing a damp bathing suit may trigger one. Many women have different tricks for avoiding yeast infections. The most popular ones include: eating yogurt, taking *L. Acidophilus* supplements, wearing cotton underwear, and cutting back on sugar.

Signs and symptoms: A yeast infection can be present inside the vagina or around the outside of the vagina. The infected area may burn, itch, and feel generally uncomfortable. Sometimes a woman's discharge is thicker than usual, has a "yeasty" smell, and may look like cottage cheese.

Treatment: Pharmacies sell over-the-counter yeast infection medications that come in one-day, three-day, and seven-day varieties—be warned, however, that some women find the one-day medication to be very irritating to their vagina and prefer the three-day alternative. Yeast infections can also be treated with a prescription pill after a diagnosis is made at a doctor's office. Since yeast infections can be fairly common and have very distinct symptoms, it's understandable that you may not want to go to the doctor every time your daughter has one. If you choose to buy an over-the-counter medication to treat the infection at home, make sure that all of the symptoms are gone after the treatment is finished. If they aren't, definitely have your daughter see a doctor to determine if something else is wrong.

URINARY TRACT INFECTIONS

What it is: A Urinary Tract Infection, or bladder infection, occurs when bacteria (often *E. coli*) enter the urethra and begin to move up the urinary tract. Again, if you are a woman, you've likely experienced one of these at some point in your life.

What causes it: Any action that might spread *E. coli* bacteria from around the anus to the urethra can cause a urinary tract infection. Although that action is often some sort of sex act, urinary tract infections can happen to women who are not sexually active as well. To help prevent urinary tract infections it's important that young women are taught to wipe from front to back. Also, they should be told to always try to pee after any sex act—which will help wash out any bacteria that might have gotten pushed into their urethra.

Signs and symptoms: Urinary tract infections are generally extremely uncomfortable, although some can be more minor. The telltale signs are feeling the need to pee constantly—even if very little or nothing comes out—and a burning sensation when actually peeing. Some people also have a fever, pain in their lower abdomen, and possibly blood in their urine. Symptoms can come on very rapidly, and the infection can spread to the kidneys if it's not treated.

Treatment: Urinary tract infections can be cured with antibiotics that a doctor can prescribe after diagnosing the infection. The antibiotics work very fast, and within twelve hours much of the discomfort will be gone. While waiting for a doctor's appointment or for the antibiotics to take effect, you can buy Uristat (or a generic version) to help ease your daughter's pain. The only side effect is that the pills will make her pee turn bright orange, something you may want to warn her about.

It's important to understand that Uristat does not cure a urinary tract infection, it just masks the pain. Even if her pain is temporarily relieved she must get in to see a doctor as soon as possible before the infection spreads to her kidneys.

BACTERIAL VAGINOSIS

What it is: Bacterial vaginosis is the overgrowth of bacteria in the vagina. For women of childbearing age, it is actually the most common vaginal infection.

What causes it: Similar to yeast infections, there isn't one cause of bacterial vaginosis. It does, however, seem to be associated with douching and having sex with someone new or with multiple people. All of those activities may upset the natural balance of vaginal bacteria. Using a condom during sex, limiting sex partners, and refraining from douching all seem to help prevent bacterial vaginosis infections. Although bacterial vaginosis is considered more of a vaginal infection than an STD, it can be spread between two female sex partners.

Signs and symptoms: The main sign of bacterial vaginosis is a fishy, foul-smelling odor coming from the vagina (that tends to get worse after sex). Other signs may include an itchy vaginal area or a burning sensation when peeing.

Treatment: Once diagnosed, bacterial vaginosis can be cured with antibiotics. If left untreated it may go away on its own, but it can also causes complications with pregnancy or any vaginal surgery or procedure, and it may make a woman more likely to contract HIV and other STDs.

TRICHOMONIASIS

What it is: Trichomoniasis is actually the most common curable sexually transmitted disease in women. Although it can also affect men, many classify it as a vaginal infection rather than an STD. Trichomoniasis is a parasite that infects a woman's vagina and can also infect a man's urethra.

What causes it: Someone can contract trichomoniasis by having vaginal sex with someone who is infected (or two women rubbing their vaginas together). Using a condom will greatly reduce the transmission of this infection.

Signs and symptoms: After someone contracts trichomoniasis, he or she may experience symptoms within a few days to a month. Although many men experience no symptoms at all, some may have an irritated penis, a slight burning when peeing or ejaculating, or notice a light discharge. Women who are infected with trichomoniasis are more likely to experience symptoms, but not all do. Those who do may notice a frothy greenish or yellowish discharge that may smell particularly strong. They may also feel pain when having sex or peeing or be generally itchy or irritated in or around their vaginal area.

Treatment: Once diagnosed, trichomoniasis can be cured through a dose of four pills. Since it is sexually transmitted, it's important that both partners get treated and test negative before continuing to have sex.

APPENDIX B: HELPFUL RESOURCES

General Sexual Health Resources

Planned Parenthood
www.plannedparenthood.com

The National Campaign to Prevent
Teen and Unplanned Pregnancy
www.thenationalcampaign.org

Afraid to Ask
www.afraidtoask.com

Advocates for Youth
www.advocatesforyouth.org

Choice USA
www.choiceusa.com

Sexuality Information and Education
Council of the United State
www.siecus.org

Dr. Katharine O'Connell White's Blog
www.gynotalk.com

General Sexual Health Information for Teens

American Social Health Association's Teen Site
www.iwannaknow.org

Planned Parenthood's Teen Site
www.teenwire.com

The National Campaign to Prevent Teen
and Unplanned Pregnancy's Teen Site
www.stayteen.org

Sex Education by Teens for Teens
www.sexetc.org

Scarleteen: Sex Education for the Real World
www.scarleteen.com

Center for Young Women's Health
www.youngwomenshealth.org

Talking with Your Kids

Talking with Kids about Tough Issues
www.talkingwithkids.org

Mothers' Voices
www.mothersvoices.org

Sexually Transmitted Diseases (STDs)

American Social Health Association
www.ashastd.org

Centers for Disease Control and Prevention
www.cdc.gov/std

Relationship Violence

The National Domestic Violence Hotline
1-800-799-SAFE (7233)
www.ndvh.org

National Youth Violence Prevention Resource Center
www.safeyouth.org

Sexual Assault

Rape, Abuse & Incest National Network
www.rainn.org

National Sexual Assault Hotline
1-800-656-HOPE (4673)

Eating Disorders

National Eating Disorders Association
www.nationaleatingdisorders.org

Alliance for Eating Disorders Awareness
www.eatingdisorderinfo.org

Sexual Orientation

Parents, Family and Friends of Lesbians & Gays
www.pflag.org

Gay, Lesbian, Bisexual and Transgender National Help Center
1-888-843-4564
www.glnh.org

BIBLIOGRAPHY

Alford S. *Science and Success, Second Edition: Programs That Work to Prevent Teen Pregnancy, HIV & Sexually Transmitted Infections.* Washington, DC: Advocates for Youth, 2008.

Blake, S.M., Ledsky, R., Goodenow, C., Sawyer, R., Lohrmann, D., & Windsor, R. "Condom Availability Programs in Massachusetts High Schools: Relationships with Condom Use and Sexual Behavior." *American Journal of Public Health* 93 (2003): 955-962.

Brown, J. *Parent Brochure: Teen Media: Mass Media and Adolescent Health.* Chapel Hill: University of North Carolina at Chapel Hill School of Journalism and Mass Communication, 2005.

Cates, J.R., Herndon, N.L., Schulz, S.L., and Darroch, J.E. *Our Voices, Our Lives, Our Futures: Youth and Sexually Transmitted Diseases.* Chapel Hill: University of North Carolina at Chapel Hill School of Journalism and Mass Communication, 2004.

Centers for Disease Control and Prevention. *HIV/AIDS Surveillance Report, 2006.* Atlanta: Centers for Disease Control and Prevention, 2008.

Centers for Disease Control and Prevention. *New Analysis Provides More Detailed Picture of Population Living With Undiagnosed HIV Infection in the United States: Suggests Significant Gaps in Knowledge of Infection across Multiple Risk, Racial, and Age Groups.* Atlanta: Centers for Disease Control and Prevention, 2009.

Centers for Disease Control and Prevention. "Chlamydia Fact Sheet." *www.cdc.gov/STD/chlamydia/STDFact-Chlamydia.htm* (accessed November 8, 2009).

Darroch, J.E., Landry, D.J., and Oslak, S. "Age Differences Between Sexual Partners in the United States." *Family Planning Perspectives* 31(1999): 160–167.

The Guttmacher Institute. "In Brief: Facts on Sex Education in the United States." New York: The Guttmacher Institute, 2006.

Hust, S., Brown, J.D., & L'Engle, K. "Boys Will be Boys and Girls Better be Prepared: An Analysis of the Rare Sexual Health Messages in Young Adolescents' Media." *Mass Communication and Society* 11 (2008): 1–21.

Kaiser Family Foundation and Seventeen Magazine. *SexSmarts.* Menlo Park: Kaiser Family Foundation, 2000.

Kaiser Family Foundation. *Sex Smarts. Communication: A Series of National Surveys of Teens about Sex.* 2002. Menlo Park: Kaiser Family Foundation, 2000.

Kirby, D. *Emerging Answers 2007: Research Findings on Programs to Reduce Teen Pregnancy and Sexually Transmitted Diseases.* Washington, DC: The National Campaign to Prevent Teen and Unplanned Pregnancy, 2007.

Liz Claiborne Inc. *Study on Teen Dating Abuse*. Teenage Research Unlimited, 2005.

Lopez, L.M., Grimes, D.A., Gallo, M.F., and Schulz, K.F. *Skin Patch and Vaginal Ring Versus Combined Oral Contraceptives for Contraception*. The Cochrane Collaboration: Cochrane Reviews, 2008.

The National Campaign to Prevent Teen and Unplanned Pregnancy. *Risky Business: A 2000 Poll: Teens Tell Us What They Really Think of Contraception and Sex.* Washington, DC: The National Campaign to Prevent Teen and Unplanned Pregnancy, 2000.

The National Campaign to Prevent Teen and Unplanned Pregnancy. *With One Voice 2002: America's Adults and Teens Sounds Off about Teen Pregnancy*. Washington, DC: The National Campaign to Prevent Teen and Unplanned Pregnancy, 2002.

The National Campaign to Prevent Teen and Unplanned Pregnancy. *Science Says: Teens and Oral Sex.* Washington, DC: The National Campaign to Prevent Teen and Unplanned Pregnancy, 2005.

The National Campaign to Prevent Teen and Unplanned Pregnancy. *With One Voice 2007: America's Adults and Teens Sounds Off About Teen Pregnancy*. Washington DC: The National Campaign to Prevent Teen and Unplanned Pregnancy, 2007.

RAINN: Rape, Abuse, and Incest National Network. "Statistics." *www.rainn.org/statistics* (accessed November 9, 2009).

The Renfrew Center Foundation for Eating Disorders. *Eating Disorders 101 Guide: A Summary of Issues, Statistics and Resources*. The Renfrew Center, 2002.

Saewyc, E.M. *et al.* "Sexual Intercourse, Abuse and Pregnancy Among Adolescent Women: Does Sexual Orientation Make a Difference?" *Family Planning Perspectives* 31 (1999): 127–31.

Salazar, L.F. *et al.* "Self-Concept and Adolescents—Refusal of Unprotected Sex: A Test of Mediating Mechanisms Among African American Girls." *Prevention Science* 5 (2004): 137–212

St. Jude Children's Research Hospital. "5 Year Cancer Survival Rates: 1962 vs. Present." *www.stjude.org* (accessed November 9, 2009).

UNAIDS. *Report on the Global AIDS Epidemic*. Geneva: UNAIDS, 2008.

Weinstock, H. *et al.* "Sexually Transmitted Diseases Among American Youth: Incidence and Prevalence Estimates, 2000." *Perspectives on Sexual and Reproductive Health* 36 (2004): 6–10.

Youth Risk Behavior Survey 2007. Atlanta: Centers for Disease Control and Prevention, 2007.

INDEX

ABOUT THE AUTHOR

Amber Madison graduated from Tufts University in 2005, where she wrote a popular sex column and studied human sexuality through a double major in Community Health and American Studies. Shortly after graduating, she finished her first book, *Hooking Up: A Girl's All-Out Guide to Sex and Sexuality* (Prometheus Books 2006), for high school and college-age young women about sexual health, sexuality, and relationships. Since then, she's traveled around the country speaking with teens and adults about sex and relationships. In 2008 she won a sexual health communication award from Choice USA.

Amber has written about sex for *Glamour* magazine, and is the sex expert for BettyConfidential.com. She has been written about by *Cosmopolitan*, *USA Today*, *U.S. News and World Report*, the *Boston Globe*, and many other publications. She's frequently quoted in newspapers, magazines, and national media such as: *Seventeen*, *Cosmopolitan*, *Men's Health*, *Newsweek*, *U.S. News and World Report*, and *USA Today*. Amber has appeared on *The Today Show*, *MTV News*, and NPR, and is a regular guest on local radio and TV newscasts. She lives in New York City.